GENE

Dr Sanjay Borude is a pioneering surgeon in obesity surgery in India. He had the privilege of learning about obesity surgery at renowned centres in the US, Belgium and Spain. He began his practice in 1989 as a general surgeon and later, from 2000, started conducting bariatric surgeries in India at Breach Candy Hospital, Mumbai. Today, Dr Borude is a super specialist in this field, specializing in lap-band, sleeve gastrectomy and gastric bypass surgeries. He has successfully treated more than 8000 morbidly obese patients to date. Dr Borude entered the *Limca Book of Records* for performing 'bariatric surgery on an 11-month-old baby'. He also holds the distinction of having performed Asia's first 'Google Eye' bariatric surgery with the Google team. He is professor emeritus at Sion Municipal Hospital and other BMC Hospitals. This is his first book.

ADVANCE PRAISE FOR THE BOOK

'Obesity is not only a health hazard but a huge setback emotionally and mentally. To deal with such a sensitive issue that can have damaging outcomes requires a relentless journey of expertise, an in-depth balance and grasp to sensitively handle the patient's distress and educate the family towards an environment conducive to promoting a healthy childhood. This book highlights that we should not take weight gain as a sign of a "happy child"; do not encourage it as a benchmark for a "healthy child". We need to break these shackles and emerge as responsible parents. Dr Sanjay Borude, a dynamic, driven surgeon and an authority on this subject has come out with a book which will be etched as a guiding light for eternity. The book touches upon all the issues that a child faces, and how the family can prevent them and help the future generation overcome these hurdles. I stand eternally grateful to Dr Sanjay Borude for dedicating his life to this issue, and I look forward to a healthy society. Our children are the future of our nation; we need to set the standards today!'—Raj Thackeray, politician and chairperson of the Maharashtra Navnirman Sena (MNS)

'*Generation XL* expertly tackles the sensitive subject of obesity, in a reader-friendly, informative style. A must-read for all—not just people dealing with weight issues. Parents of young children dealing with weight gain and related health problems will benefit greatly from Dr Sanjay Borude's well-researched book, in which he describes obesity as a "time bomb"'—Shobhaa De, novelist and columnist

'When Dr Sanjay Borude came to meet me, he told me he was a fan of mine. But after we met, I turned into a fan of his! He sings and he's an artiste, so when he does his surgeries, I have no doubts he must be doing it artistically. He has been a doctor for the past thirty years. Initially he used to perform surgeries on cancer patients. Later, he realized he could serve humanity even better by tackling the issue of child obesity. I can say this from my own experience. I was overweight and would feel dejected and upset because of that. I had a lot of difficulty losing weight. Children who are either born obese or those who turn obese because of what their parents feed them face difficulties all their lives. Dr Sanjay Borude has done tremendous work in this area. Consider this: he has even carried out a surgery on an 11-month-old infant, and she is now a healthy 12-year-old. When I look around, I see parents giving their children all sorts to things to eat—three to four ice creams at a time, sandwiches with thick layers of cheese and what not. If, instead of that, children ate the satvik, native foods our parents gave us and if they ate only so much as would fit into a palm, it would be sufficient. That's what Dr Borude says, and I too am saying this, because Dr Borude is a splendid doctor, and he sings nicely as well. In my view, Dr Sanjay Borude is the best doctor in the world. He's also a very good human being. Where needed, he works for free and saves people's lives. Can there be a greater thing than saving lives? We cannot see God but we can see doctors, and for me, Dr Sanjay Borude is God!'—Asha Bhosle, playback singer

'The book discusses the genesis and management of childhood obesity with all the relevant details. Obesity in children is a preventable problem with very few exceptions. Prevention should start from birth with exclusive breastfeeding for the first six months followed by complementary feeds from the family pot, while breastfeeding is continued for at least another six months. Of course, it must be subsequently maintained with a good lifestyle. This can happen only if health is monitored by a growth chart so that mild weight gain can be picked up and corrected. It is not only the weight but also height and BMI. This is a health card similar to a progress card in school. Indian Academy of Pediatrics has published growth charts for Indian boys and girls, and the chart is modified in a simple way to give BMI on the same chart that depicts weight and height, and it can show whether the child is underweight, overweight or obese. These charts can be downloaded for free from IAP's website'—Dr Yeshwant K. Amdekar, paediatrician

GENERATION
XL

Tackling and Preventing
Childhood Obesity in India

DR SANJAY BORUDE

ONE OF INDIA'S LEADING BARIATRIC SURGEONS

EBURY
PRESS

An imprint of Penguin Random House

EBURY PRESS

USA | Canada | UK | Ireland | Australia
New Zealand | India | South Africa | China

Ebury Press is part of the Penguin Random House group of companies
whose addresses can be found at global.penguinrandomhouse.com

Published by Penguin Random House India Pvt. Ltd
4th Floor, Capital Tower 1, MG Road,
Gurugram 122 002, Haryana, India

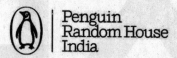

Penguin
Random House
India

First published in Ebury Press by Penguin Random House India 2022

Copyright © Dr Sanjay Borude 2022

All rights reserved

10 9 8 7 6 5 4 3 2 1

The views and opinions expressed in this book are the author's own and the
facts are as reported by him which have been verified to the extent possible,
and the publishers are not in any way liable for the same.

ISBN 9780143441816

Typeset in Adobe Caslon Pro by MAP Systems, Bengaluru, India
Printed at Replika Press Pvt. Ltd, India

This book is sold subject to the condition that it shall not, by way of trade
or otherwise, be lent, resold, hired out, or otherwise circulated without the
publisher's prior consent in any form of binding or cover other than that in
which it is published and without a similar condition including this condition
being imposed on the subsequent purchaser.

www.penguin.co.in

To Zoya Khan

Contents

Part 3

Prologue

If a list of the most commonly used words is compiled under the spectrum of health and wellness, weight would definitely figure prominently on it. Almost everyone, irrespective of their gender or age, frets about the calories they consume or the inches they could add to their waistline with a single meal. And, if not about their own weight, there is always the worry of a parent, spouse or child gaining kilograms they shouldn't. It wouldn't be wrong to say that weight is perhaps one of the most stress-inducing words of our times.

Unfortunately, most people obsess about their weight for cosmetic reasons. In Indian society, parents fear that their daughter won't get that coveted alliance if she is overweight. Many youngsters believe being successful and being overweight are mutually exclusive. They ignore the fact that some of the world's highest earning entertainers, such as Oprah Winfrey, have struggled with those extra kilos.

It's important to get scientific about weight and its associated problems. Modern medicine has—in the last few decades—proved beyond a doubt that weight is not inversely proportional to looks but to overall health. There is enough research to indicate that being overweight or obese is akin to issuing an open invitation to ill-health. It is a risk factor for diseases such as hypertension, diabetes, stroke, coronary artery diseases and cancer, among many others.

As a bariatric surgeon who has counselled and treated a spectrum of patients with weight issues including people from varying socio-economic groups over the last two decades, I have noticed an emerging dimension in the obesity problem. Children today weigh more than those from the previous generations. A cursory look at the playgrounds of most schools in urban areas would reveal children looking a tad bit heavier than they should be for their age. Research has shown how students in the 13–16 age group from suburban Mumbai took nearly 2000 steps less than their counterparts in the UK.

In terms of weight, it would be apt to label today's children and youth as Generation XL. The wiry frame that one associated with Indian children until a few decades ago has made way for an overgrown, size XL-wearing teenager.

However, all is not lost. There are ways—ranging from lifestyle modifications and diets to bariatric surgery—that could help control this public health problem of obesity. This book will capture how acute the obesity problem is among our children and, more importantly, enumerate constructive ways to tackle it.

The main reason behind writing this book is to create awareness about the dangers of obesity, not only for an individual but for society as a whole.

There is an urgent need to educate every parent, grandparent, teacher, nanny and guardian about the medical fact that a chubby baby isn't really a healthy baby. It has to be impressed upon them that chubbiness could just be the first indication of obesity—a tell-tale sign, right in infancy, that generations of Indians have wrongly associated with good health. Chubbiness could be an indicator of a high calorific diet that isn't a good thing. Moreover, there are enough research-based studies in India to bust the myth that a chubby baby grows up to be a robust and healthy individual. It would be equally wrong to presume that a lean child will grow up to be malnourished and unhealthy.

The only reality in terms of nutrition is that India is becoming a nation of obese individuals; our children are 'sizes' bigger than what we were at their age. It has been estimated after careful study that obesity affects 2.2 billion children and adults worldwide, which amounts to nearly one in three people. Around 40 per cent of this obese population of the world lives in India.

Doctors and nutritionists have talked about the ticking obesity time bomb for over a decade now. But their efforts were perhaps too local, and not universal enough, to become a movement.

There are many misleading advertisements that talk about quick fixes, over-the-counter weight loss products and lifestyle gurus who promise a 'healthy you' with the shortest turnaround. None of them talk about the intelligent and easy choice of ensuring that one only needs to tuck in adequate calories and exercise regularly while ensuring adequate mental and physical rest.

To borrow from Greek scientist and philosopher Aristotle's Golden Mean rule, moderation—especially in diet or in food portions—is always the best.

We need to educate our children about the need to satiate their appetite with small, multiple and nutritious meals. We need to tell them to give their fingers some rest from constant online gaming and motivate them to get on to the playground. Perhaps, parents could innovate and come up with a cheat code, an immensely popular word with gaming enthusiasts. Let us urge them to put in thirty minutes of extra physical activity and qualify for a cheat day. This could include a home-made burger using fresh ingredients as opposed to gorging on a patty that was frozen for six months before being fried to that familiar processed taste within seconds.

We have to accept that Generation XL is the new public health threat to our society and work towards bringing the unhealthy situation under control. The anti-obesity movement now needs a collaborative effort between the government, schools, the healthcare sector, the food and beverage industries and the fourth estate. Awareness about obesity and its crippling side-effects need to be reiterated at every level so that people imbibe the lessons and make healthy changes to their lifestyle.

Introduction

As I walk up to the stage in the air-conditioned auditorium of a posh, suburban Mumbai school, (like many other schools I visit) I take a mandatory quick look around. Parents, mostly mothers in their thirties and forties, are assembled for the Parent-Teacher meeting that has been organized by the school authorities. They typically invite a guest speaker like me who will give a talk on a health-related subject. I am here to talk about childhood obesity.

Body Mass Index (BMI)

BMI is calculated by dividing weight in kilograms by height in metres squared (kg/m).

Status	BMI (kg/m²)
Too thin for their height	<18.5
Normal	18.5–24.9
Overweight	25.0–29.9
Obese	>30

BMI is a global tool commonly used by doctors to access health and health-related standards. As shown in the table above, based on your BMI score, you are categorized under various categories such as normal, overweight or obese.

As I glance around, I see very few parents who look fit according to our medical standards—with an appropriate BMI that indicates a healthy amount of body fat. Most are overweight and some are even obese. And some, despite their healthy weight, seem fatigued. Being a bariatric surgeon, the causes and consequences of this silent killer—obesity—flash across my mind. Throughout my practice, I have noticed that we Indians are often conflicted between traditional and global—be it in values or cuisines. Secondly, with the advent of both technology and urbanization, lifestyles have undergone a sea change—physical activity has diminished and we have adapted to incorrect food habits. Moreover, we have abandoned a healthy relationship with food, and developed an unhealthy one with consumerism instead.

Like many countries across the world that are fighting to keep this epidemic at bay, India too has been a part of the battle. As much as obesity is a public health concern, I strongly believe that the change and the real war begins at home.

The key is awareness—not only about how to tackle obesity, but also about how to prevent it. In only about 25 per cent of total cases is obesity caused due to genetic reasons. In most cases, it is the consequence of the lifestyle adopted. It is at home that we develop most of the habits of our adult life. It is also at home that children emulate adults and their beliefs, which affects their relationship with food and the environment. This is why I know that, time and again, we need to talk about 'childhood obesity' with parents as well as children.

As the years roll by, the dangers of this epidemic are becoming more and more acute. And as a bariatric surgeon, I feel surgery is not the resort for childhood obesity. Thus, for the past couple of years, creating awareness has formed a big part of my practice. My book is an extension of all the awareness programmes that my team and I have been conducting.

The book is divided into three sections: awareness about the disease, managing the condition and bariatric surgery, the final choice. The book is intended to be a parent-child read; illustrations, tables, charts, etc., are included for the child, as it increases their awareness about food, calories, exercise and so on.

I hope this book will help you understand how serious a threat obesity poses to our lives, and to the lives of our children, and how we can combat it from an immediate, personal level that translates to fighting the larger threat.

Part 1

Part I

Chapter 1

The Obesity Time Bomb

India has the second highest number of obese children in the world, with 14.4 million reported cases, according to a new study published in *The New England Journal of Medicine*.[1] The country is the second most populous nation in the world with 27.05 per cent of its population in the 0–14 age range. The obesity rank corresponds to India's global position in terms of population, but the numbers are alarming nonetheless.

Developing countries, such as India, have a unique problem of a double burden wherein one end of the spectrum comprises of obesity in children and adolescents while the other encompasses malnutrition

---

[1] Prajwal Bhat, 'India has the second highest number of obese children in the world', https://www.downtoearth.org.in/news/health/india-has-the-second-higest-number-of-obese-children-in-the-world-58115.

and underweight individuals. Childhood obesity is a forerunner of metabolic syndrome, poor physical health, mental disorders, respiratory problems and glucose intolerance, all of which can continue into adulthood.

With the widespread invasion of fast-food chains—especially American and Chinese—we are at the forefront of childhood obesity with only a marginal difference in its incidence between urban and rural Indians.

Data point 1: Nearly every fifth child in school could be unhealthy.

A recent study (2017) published in *The Indian Journal of Endocrinology and Metabolism* identified that 18–21 per cent of Indian teens (in the 13–18 age group) in urban schools are overweight or obese.[2]

Data point 2: India is home to 14.4 million obese children and is second only to China which has 15.3 million obese children.

Every parent believes that the neighbours' child is fat while their own is healthy. Being 'healthy' is not a mere linguistic misinterpretation, but also a cultural one.

---

[2] Harish Ranjani et al., 'Epidemiology of childhood overweight and obesity in India: A systematic review', https://www.ncbi.nlm.nih.gov/pmc/articles/PMC4859125/.

Data point 3: In India, adolescents from parts of Punjab, Maharashtra, Delhi and South India are overweight and obese (11–29 per cent).

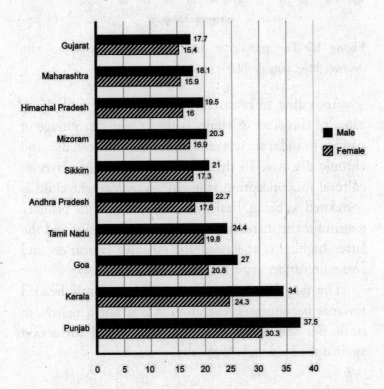

Figure 1.1 The top ten states in India in order of percentage of obese people, with Punjab representing the maximum overweight population.[3]

---

[3] Based on data from the 2007 National Family Health Survey.

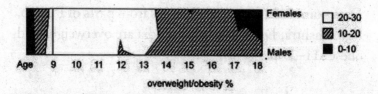

Figure 1.2 The prevalence and percentage of children with overweight/obesity problems between the ages 0–18.

According to research, the most potent underlying cause of this state of affairs is that a high percentage of parents in India are unaware of the link between diet and chronic diseases. To this, one can add another layer of cultural misconception whereby an overweight child is correlated as being 'healthy'. The former is the primary reason for the increasing occurrences of obesity, and the latter highlights the need for effective education and communication.

The fact that the next generation is firmly headed towards becoming 'Generation XL' is not a reason to smile but should be seen as a clarion call for action against the epidemic of obesity.

Causes of Obesity

It is commonly believed that obesity arises due to eating junk, unhealthy food, fried in saturated fat, etc.—the list is endless.

But social and cultural factors are equally responsible and often unaccounted for. The paucity of playgrounds in urban areas leads to children being glued to screens with little physical activity. Their day is packed with extracurricular activities and tuitions, leaving no time or energy for play. Physical activity becomes minimal or is missing from daily schedules unless obesity or its symptoms arise.

Exercise is often perceived or undertaken as a measure to combat obesity. Many forget that physical activity is important for sound physiological, mental and overall well-being irrespective of whether the person is overweight or otherwise.

However, before we steer towards preventive or curative measures, we need to understand obesity.

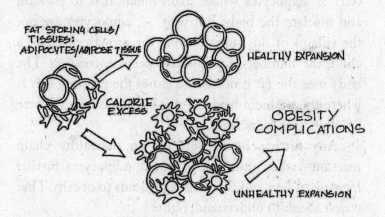

Looks Complicated?

Cancer is easily explained: uncontrolled multiplication of non-functional or improper cells.

In a similar fashion, obesity is the unhealthy expansion of fat storing cells to accommodate all the extras that our children are consuming without sweating or burning them out.

Everything Begins at a Cellular Level . . . Alas!

How we wish we could just keep eating like Kung Fu Panda and still be a 'Dragon Warrior', don't we?

Let us first understand the molecular or basic mechanism of obesity. The body contains many types of tissues. The ones we are interested in are known as fat cells or adipocytes whose main function is to cushion and insulate the body. But wait . . . adipocytes are not the villains of this story. During the growth phase of a child, the number of adipocytes keeps increasing. The body uses the fat it needs and stores the rest, but this is where the problem begins—this storage causes the size of adipocytes to increase.

Any further intake sets off an unhealthy chain reaction—when more fat is stored, adipocytes further increase in size, and this ultimately leads to obesity. That wasn't tough to understand, right?

Weight loss programmes, therefore, could help decrease the size of these adipocytes but not their numbers. This means that once a person is obese, they need to continue weight loss exercises for life to avoid an increase in the size of adipocytes.

Emotional Context of Food in India

India is the land of many things, including food. Beyond nutrition, it is a source of comfort, nostalgia, mental wellness and celebrations. With time, festivals have also transpired as occasions to indulge in celebratory meals wherein food plays a huge role. For instance, there is a lot of indulgence in sweets during festivals like Diwali and Christmas. When on a fast, people are encouraged to consume high-calorie or high-carbohydrate foods.

Food is also an emotional anchor. Fried goodies are associated with the rains while winters call for rich, greasy fare. Recipes from grandmothers' and mothers' kitchens have nostalgic value and often become comfort food. This emphasizes the importance of food as nourishment, as celebration and as a way of living among Indians.

Dieting, fasting and other adapted dietary habits are also celebrated in modern India and have found space along with a side dish of exercise and yoga. We are a food-loving community and obesity is a result of this love. Often, genes also predispose individuals to obesity.

While obesity is not a crime or an individual flaw, it is a silent, and sometimes violent, killer as it is associated with a number of diseases. Figure 1.3 should help us understand this better.

COMPLICATIONS OF CHILDHOOD OBESITY

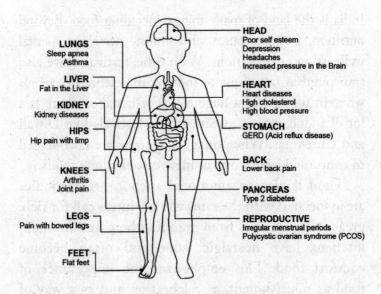

LUNGS
Sleep apnea
Asthma

LIVER
Fat in the Liver

KIDNEY
Kidney diseases

HIPS
Hip pain with limp

KNEES
Arthritis
Joint pain

LEGS
Pain with bowed legs

FEET
Flat feet

HEAD
Poor self esteem
Depression
Headaches
Increased pressure in the Brain

HEART
Heart diseases
High cholesterol
High blood pressure

STOMACH
GERD (Acid reflux disease)

BACK
Lower back pain

PANCREAS
Type 2 diabetes

REPRODUCTIVE
Irregular menstrual periods
Polycystic ovarian syndrome (PCOS)

The consequences of obesity range from general health issues to heart problems to poor self-esteem. It is critical to check this generation's march towards XL and the plus size. If obesity catches up with them at a younger age, ailments will affect children earlier than they did for the previous generations. There is an urgent need to draw up a plan to check increasing obesity rates among children. But first, we need to identify the root cause.

For the last two decades, India has been termed as a 'fast growing economy'. What are its implications on obesity? As per a report in the *Indian Journal of Medical Research*, 'We are in the middle of major epidemiological, nutritional and demographic transitions that tend to promote obesity in all age groups.' But when one looks at the prevalence of obesity alone, there is no clear, secular trend.

So Why Is Childhood Obesity on the Rise?

It is increasingly being recognized that parents' perception of their child's weight is an important factor in planning public health interventions to reduce the prevalence of obesity.[4]

I understand that being a parent, especially a first-time one, is serious business, which one undertakes without prior experience. We all try to do our best for our children. Many studies have revealed that parents fail to correctly gauge that their children are overweight. In several cases, parents also fail to recognize early symptoms of obesity. In case of a diagnosis, parents should first understand the determinants of obesity before embarking on the journey of diet/exercise and medication and seek appropriate help from their doctor.

It is extremely important to have a 360-degree view of the causative factors of your child's obesity even though, more often than not, a sedentary lifestyle and dietary habits top the list. Figure 1.4 puts together a comprehensive list of factors affecting childhood obesity.

---

[4] Harish Ranjani et al., 'Epidemiology of childhood overweight and obesity in India: A systematic review', https://www.ncbi.nlm.nih.gov/pmc/articles/PMC4757535/.

DETERMINANTS OF PEDIATRIC OBESITY

- Physical activity
- Sleep
- Screen/sedentary time

Energy expenditure

- Genetics
- Epigenetics
- Ethnicity
- Country of birth
- Birth weight
- BMI rebound

PEDIATRIC OBESITY

- Endocrine disease
- Hypothalamic damage
- Medications
- Socioeconomic position
  Cultural/normative
  constraints
- Urban/rural residence

Energy intake

- Diet
- Family food choices

Now, let us take a closer look at Mumbai's obesity map to find a few illustrative answers regarding the state of obesity in the region. In 2010, doctors from a medical school in south Mumbai visited four schools to study the prevalence of obesity among their students. Two of the chosen schools were privately run and located in affluent areas in the city, while the other two were run by the municipal corporation with children hailing from less affluent economic backgrounds going there to study. From this study, it was observed that more boys than girls were overweight or obese. Secondly, children in the private schools were significantly heavier than those in government schools.

Clearly, we could all have guessed the result. But what interested me was that the affluent families are more educated compared to the families of children studying in municipal schools. With more access to resources and information, the former should have healthier habits. But assumptions, even if logical, are not facts. This also highlighted the gender difference in the incidence of obesity among children.

Obesity is accompanied by a plethora of diseases as mentioned. After understanding the consequences or rather the companion diseases of obesity, it is important for parents to know the reason(s) for obesity among children.

Food

Food is perceived as the primary reason of obesity but it is not food per se that is the problem. The type of food a child consumes, portions served on their plate, the consumption of high-calorie snacks and/or colas and, their attitude towards food form the crux of the matter. It is high time that we revert to our healthy Indian diets rather than adopt the popular cuisine of fast foods. Socio-economic status also has significant implications for obesity risk as it increases spending capacity.

Lack of Physical Activity

The next important culprit that adds kilos to the scale is low or absolute lack of physical activity.

Along with these major contributing factors, we should also be aware of the role played by genetic make-up and hormonal imbalances that leave only surgery as the main, viable option for obesity treatment. Parental obesity is considered a stronger predictor of obesity in adulthood than the child's weight status at less than 3 years of age. There are genetic factors that can influence the susceptibility of a given child to an obesity-conducive environment.[5]

It is also observed in a few studies that family incomes also play an important role in constituting the child's obesity.

Some studies say that being breastfed for longer than six months reduce the chances of a child becoming overweight later in life by about 20 to 40 per cent. Others suggest that excessive non-vegetarian food can also be problematic, since the excess protein from meat, if not burned through exercise, is deposited as fat. In my own research in adult patients, this was found to be untrue.

A commonsensical answer would be that obesity results from an imbalance between the energy (calories) consumed and the calories burnt with exercise.

Technology

Another monster is the evolution of technology. In an era where gaming consoles and computer games are

---

[5] Claude Bouchard, 'Childhood obesity: Are genetic differences involved?', https://www.ncbi.nlm.nih.gov/pmc/articles/PMC2677002/.

found practically in every house, children don't get an opportunity to burn the calories they consume. They sit hunched up in front of their consoles or study tables instead of running around on playgrounds. However, between diet and exercise, research has shown that diets are far more important in weight loss than exercise. While physical activity is a great complementary measure, the focus must remain on consuming whole foods that are low on calories but provide ample nutrition. It takes half-an-hour of running to burn 300 calories, but two minutes or less to consume them.

Speaking of consuming fewer calories, a typical Indian school child in an urban setting is likely to carry two lunch boxes to school. As working parents are unlikely to have time to cook fresh food every day, chances are that at least one box would have ready-to-eat high-calorie packaged foods like chips, biscuits, cakes, etc. Once back home, the child will eat a meal before playing digital games or finishing homework. This sedentariness that has crept into every child's life is one of the biggest culprits in the obesity epidemic. Combine this with junk food and the obesity puzzle seems almost complete.

As per the *Indian Journal of Medical Research*, 'Low levels of physical activity are definitely promoted by an automated and automobile-oriented environment that is conducive to a sedentary lifestyle. Community design and infrastructure characteristics are also becoming increasingly important in determining levels of obesity in populations. Such factors include availability of safe walkways, bicycle paths, playgrounds and other avenues for physical activity-related recreation.'[6]

Parenting and Obesity

There are many social and emotional factors that contribute to childhood obesity. While genetics does play a key role, some studies show that it is the culprit in less than 5 per cent cases. Other related factors are excessive stress experienced by the pregnant mother, which can cause increased insulin sensitivity, leading to obesity in adulthood. The BMI of a child's parents could doom them into obesity too. It has been found that children inherit a sizeable portion of their parents' weight. This causes a vicious cycle wherein a child has a tendency to be fat due to the weight of their parents. The excess BMI of their parents likely stems from unhealthy eating habits that they themselves have succumbed to, which the child will also pick up through interactions with them. An already acquired predisposition to obesity can easily actualize the risk of obesity a child carries and cause them a lifetime of health issues.

In addition, the nature of the environment a child grows up in can also be crucial. This can include several factors like the stability of their parents' marriage,

[6] Manu Raj and R. Krishna Kumar, 'Obesity in children and adolescents', https://www.ncbi.nlm.nih.gov/pmc/articles/PMC3028965/.

whether the child has adequate friends, how involved their parents are depending on their work commitments, etc. A child needs encouragement to play outside, either from friends, since they need companions to play with, or from parents, who can communicate the importance of doing so. In the absence of any such motivation, the child will choose to stay indoors and watch television or partake in sedentary activities.

Parenting is an important factor in the obesity epidemic; a parent's willingness to experiment with healthy options could make children more accepting. Even if a child has adopted some unhealthy habits, such as eating from canteens or eating late at night, studies show that a parent's willingness to adapt and enforce changes in their child's eating behaviour is crucial to controlling their weight.

This does not imply restricting the food that the child eats, but setting a schedule for meals and providing balanced meals that are palatable and also contain the required nutrients. Palatability is especially crucial since children can refuse to eat altogether and wait for opportunities when they have access to different foods— from a peer's tiffin at school, eateries near their campus, etc.

It is imperative for parents to set the right relationship between the child and food. Leniency will result in eating excessively and obesity, whereas severe restrictions can be detrimental. In light of this, parents must take the extra effort of cooking meals that are healthy but seem appetizing at the same time. Many of these meals can be made with minimal resources, and, usually do not need much time to prepare. The effort lies in finding appropriate recipes and routinizing the entire process.

Besides food itself, other factors need to be accounted for as well. If children are allowed to eat in front of the television, there are higher chances of them packing in larger portions to stretch the meal break and enjoy extended television time. They may take second or third servings if the television is playing and eat mindlessly while watching their favourite shows. It is also an accepted fact that mealtime is healthier if it is a family affair.

This is not just from the viewpoint of reducing weight; eating as a family can have significant emotional benefits for all parties involved.

Research shows that children and adolescents, contrary to popular perception, prefer eating with their parents. It gives them a sense of security and makes them feel like a part of the family. Children who eat with their families regularly consume more fruits and vegetables, are happier and get better grades than those who eat alone. There are countless more benefits to eating as a family, and this is one activity parents must try to follow.[7] Parents need to lead by example as far as nutrition is concerned.

---

[7] 'Nine scientifically proven reasons to eat dinner as a family', https://www.goodnet.org/articles/9-scientifically-proven-reasons-to-eat-dinner-as-family.

As per a report in the *Indian Journal of Endocrinology and Metabolism*, a study was conducted in a school-based intervention in north India, which consisted of four groups focusing on: obesity prevention and reduction; prevention of excessive sweet, chocolate and carbohydrate consumption; reducing daily TV watching; and increasing physical activity. School children aged 5–18 years (n = 610) participated in two-hour long weekly sessions for six months. The intervention reported 0.33 per cent reduction in obesity, 27.5 per cent reduction in sweets, chocolates, and carbohydrate-rich food consumption, 17 per cent reduction in sedentary activities, and 19 per cent reduction in prolonged TV watching.[8]

Another research aimed to evaluate the impact of a school-based health and nutrition education programme on the knowledge and behaviour of 3,128 school children (8–18 years), 2,241 parents and 841 teachers from three different cities representing north India. Low baseline knowledge and behaviour scores were reported in 75–94 per cent of government and 48–78 per cent of private school children, across all age groups. However, younger children aged 8–11 years fared better than those aged 12–18 years. It was observed in another study that a higher proportion of children

---

[8] Harish Ranjani et al., 'Determinants, consequences and prevention of childhood overweight and obesity,' https://www.ncbi.nlm.nih.gov/pmc/articles/PMC4266865/.

who brought packed lunch and carried fruit to school showed marked improvements in insulin resistance, β-cell function, disposition index and sub-clinical inflammation. Similarly, a recent study from southern India revealed that a significant increase in the level of knowledge among normal and overweight children can be achieved through mass education programmes.[9]

Role of Healthcare Policies

A point raised by American entertainer Oprah Winfrey must be emphasized here—no child is fat alone. There is almost always a mechanism or a series of oversights that contribute to fatty deposition at a young age. In fact, governmental policies contribute immensely to expanding waistlines because of the government's reluctance to levy extra tax on corporate houses selling sugary beverages and fatty fried foods. Countries, such as the US and Mexico, have experimented with the introduction of 'fat tax' on sodas and fried foods, but the idea hasn't gained popularity among nations yet, even though it is increasingly being recognized as the only way ahead to stop obesity.

Some countries and states in the US have implemented a solitary soda tax, but the measures have

---

[9] Priyali Shah et al., 'Improvement in nutrition-related knowledge and behaviour of urban Asian Indian school children', https://pubmed.ncbi.nlm.nih.gov/20370939/.

backfired, mainly because taxing one item cannot make much of a difference.

In India, among healthcare policies and insurance coverage, appropriate measures are still required to highlight the dangerous role of obesity among non-communicable diseases and subsequent consequences.

As this chapter has illustrated, obesity involves many variables and legislation must account for a wider variety of foods for taxation to be effective. Furthermore, even if laws were to change adequately, they need the support of people like us to ensure their success.

The failure of local governments to provide adequate open spaces for children (and their parents) is also a culprit. Children have no place to run, play or burn the empty calories they have consumed throughout the day, resulting in them getting chubbier. Many parents of lower socio-economic backgrounds cannot afford to send their children to training academies, and parks are perhaps the only and most crucial places for their exercise.

On the emotional front, children who are depressed or suffer from anxiety disorders, gain weight due to the comfort they draw from food. These children often struggle to make friends, which leads to overeating as a coping mechanism. This creates a vicious cycle wherein food satiates the emotional void of depression leading to obesity. Soon, the child is addicted to food as a coping mechanism—food and depression fuel one another, leading to further weight gain and emotional disorders.

Morbidly obese patients who successfully lost hundreds of pounds of weight have described some sadness at what they perceived as losing a friend with whom they had built a friendship, akin to what one has with a companion.

In some cases, parents inadvertently encourage children to associate eating junk with positive feelings. Many households offer eatables (mainly chocolates or sweets) as a reward for accomplishing tasks and good behaviour may be recognized by trips to fast food joints. While even the most dedicated athletes have cheat days, using junk food as positive reinforcement sets the wrong precedent. Over time, these habits will lead to health problems.

Children don't realize the harm of overeating or its link to obesity. They fear obesity only because of the ridicule they may suffer from peers. It is our duty, as a society, to ensure that our children don't binge eat, and that they eat right and on time.

On a positive note, one only needs to remember that obesity is an easily preventable disease. Parents, despite their knowledge, may find it hard to restrain their children from eating junk, street or fast food.

The following example from a news report in *Livescience.com* may serve as a guiding light: Michelle Morton, a mother of three, stocked only healthy snacks, such as yogurt and fruits, at home so that her children had no option but to eat them when hungry. But, as her children were attracted to junk food, she designated days—Cheat Days—to eat a brownie or a cake.[10] The point being that it is fine to take a day off from healthy eating and eat what your stomach craves—as long as one compensates with additional activity the next day and gets back on track with a regular diet.

Enrolling children into sports or other physical activities helps them learn discipline and eat healthy, since unhealthy eating will inhibit their ability to compete in these sports. This gives them a healthy incentive to eat nutritious foods and eases the burden of many parents who won't have to force their children to eat healthy.

---

[10] Amanda Chan, 'Junk Food Nation: How Parents Are Ruining Kids' Health', https://www.livescience.com/14280-parents-feed-kids-junk.html.

Chapter 2

The Obese Child

Every year, the number of parents visiting my clinic for consultations for their obese children increases. When bariatric surgery started making inroads in India twenty years ago, children never visited bariatric surgeons. At the risk of repeating myself, I reiterate that the advent of liberalization has changed that, owing to the easy accessibility of ready-to-eat foods that are high in calories. The lack of open spaces for children to play and many other social reasons act as factors that result in weight gain. Currently, I receive at least one new paediatric patient in my clinic for advice each week. Parents of children as young as eighteen months have dropped by for a consultation; less than 5 per cent of them require surgical intervention.

A study giving a snapshot of physical activity and food habits among private school children in India states, 'Lifestyle changes concomitant with globalization, economic development and access to technology are often implicated in concerns related to the emergence of obesity and chronic diseases in India. New behaviours, such as eating processed foods and eating out, have been associated with obesity among children aged 5–19 years. Families are increasingly able to purchase televisions, computers and gaming systems, and children spend leisure time in sedentary activities indoors.'[11]

Emphasis on education also affects physical activity, since children spend considerable time studying. Simultaneously, changes related to globalization, economic development and technology have contributed to major improvements in health. For instance, changes in food production and prices increase the availability of energy-rich foods, addressing India's persistent problem of underweight individuals.

On 22 November 2011, I performed a bariatric surgery on an eleven-month-old child named Zoya Khan, at Mumbai's prestigious Breach Candy Hospital. She was the youngest child to undergo bariatric surgery in India. The operation stoked a debate in society, but I firmly believe I have helped the child lead a normal life,

---

[11] Shailaja S. Patil et al., 'A snapshot of physical activity and food habits among private school children in India', https://www.ncbi.nlm.nih.gov/pmc/articles/PMC5179030/.

given her genetic obesity. Much transpires within the body beyond the accumulation of fat; the excess weight can systematically destroy the body.

Check the skin of morbidly obese children and you will notice deep folds. Their hands and legs seem like stubs in comparison to their trunk. Many of them cannot fit in chairs and need broad sofas to feel comfortable. Several among them also develop a condition called tibia vara, also known as Blount's disease. The condition causes the knee bones to appear angular and bent due to excess weight on the tibia or shin bone. Their movement is restricted which, in a sense, adds to their sedentary lifestyle and worsens their weight problem, creating another vicious cycle.

Visits from such patients have a sad ring to them because these children are too young to realize that their health is at stake. As the adults discuss obesity-related problems and cures, they play with their parents' mobile or some hand-held personal gaming device. This underlines the fact that screens dominate our leisure time and the physical and mental alertness in real-time has reduced. Children increasingly opt to engage with gadgets for entertainment, and physical activity is taking a backseat in the era of development and globalization.

Parents are often motivated by external factors—the child's appearance, hostile looks their child receives from strangers, the teasing, etc. and not necessarily the implications of a bad diet on health. This reflects a poor understanding of the various dangerous effects obesity can have on a child. Weight gain and loss is common amidst growing children. But recognizing the numbers that cause ailments is crucial. The only way to raise awareness regarding this is through health programmes aimed at educating parents on the health of their children.

I have obtained permission from parents to chronicle their child's battle with obesity. It is interesting to note that none of the parents or the children can pinpoint when exactly obesity took over their lives or what it is that they were doing so wrong that weight gain never stopped. Obesity stealthily creeps into people's lives and there are seldom any alarms that can notify the exact moment when weight gain converts to an ailment. The stories are alarming, but each demonstrates that the human spirit can get around most challenges.

We cannot, of course, forget Emam Husain, the Egyptian woman who wore the unhappy crown of being the world's heaviest woman weighing around 500 kilograms. She stopped standing or walking at the age of 11. She had a genetic mutation that affected her metabolism and led to weight gain. But her story underlines why the medical field needs more research and effort to stop every form of obesity and its various contributing factors.

Obese children often tell me that other children don't want to play with them because they are too slow at a game or unable to keep pace with others while running. Such occurrences can psychologically affect them. Social stigma leads to lack of self-confidence, depression and a sense of rejection. It is said that older obese individuals who suffer from chronic depression are five times more likely to commit suicide than people who are not obese.

It is important that parents prevent their kids from reaching that stage. They can begin by underlining the need for proper nourishment to lead a mentally and physically healthy lifestyle.

Urbanization and industrialization have immensely contributed to increasing children's energy intake while decreasing their energy expenditure, thus promoting obesity. The challenge lies in formulating policies that address how best to change this built environment in a positive manner in order to maintain children's energy balance and prevent excessive weight gain.

The reluctance of policymakers to regulate the food environment is a direct consequence of the belief that people's food choices reflect their true desires. The reality is that food choices are often automatic, and, in children, they are driven by the effects of mass media, family habits and peer pressure.

In an article examining the prevalence of obesity in adolescents and children, a clear example of this influence was shown through the placement of candy/chocolates near cash registers at supermarkets. This is a widely acknowledged promotional strategy called 'impulse marketing'. The article states, 'Impulse marketing encourages spur-of-the-moment emotion-related purchases that are triggered by seeing a product or a related message. It works by placing goods at prominent locations in supermarkets. For instance, end of the aisle or at the cash counter. These are seen to account for about 30 per cent of all supermarket sales. The common belief is that those who respond to impulse marketing lack self-control and should learn how to resist such marketing strategies. But these tactics psychologically manipulate the buyer into making purchases that often include chips, sugary food and drinks. However, anyone who has visited a supermarket will know that most last-minute purchasing decisions are made quickly and automatically without substantial cognitive input.'[12]

It is important that policymakers also intervene to dismiss food advertisements with misleading messages. Instant noodles are promoted as a healthy food choice even though their main ingredient is refined wheat. They are artificially fortified with nutrients and marketed as a 'source of essential nutrition'. Health drinks, granola bars and cornflakes that are packaged as diet foods often pack in alarming quantities of sugar.

Even if the buyer is aware of misnomers that prevail in fast foods, the choice to buy fast food is impulsive. Whole foods like fruits, vegetables and whole grains require more thought. This can be attributed to the fact

---

[12] 'Determinants, consequences and prevention of childhood overweight and obesity: An Indian context', https://www.ncbi.nlm.nih.gov/pmc/articles/PMC4266865/.

that instant foods offer instant gratification. They are cheap and less tedious to prepare and consume. This, again, boils down to the responsibility of authorities to regulate what masses have access to and how nutrition can be facilitated through better policies.

Policymakers need to understand the effect of these marketing strategies—employed to increase sales—in relation to public health and limit the types of foods that can be displayed in prominent end-of-aisle locations and move foods that could promote chronic diseases to locations that are not easily accessible.

The most important step, however, is awakening the parental instinct.

Working parents in urban set-ups rely on food ordering apps and ready-to-eat meals, leading to eating disorders in children. Impulse-based eating (packaged or junk food) overrules holistic dietary choices. Bingeing, eating between meals and midnight snacking becomes prevalent. Apart from empty calories, children may consume energy drinks that contain artificial proteins and carcinogenic preservatives like aspartame. This combination of unhealthy fare affects the gut and its ability to metabolize food.

Working parents often do not have the time to supervise their children's diet. They consume microwavable semi-cooked food that has little nutritional benefit. Guilt-ridden, parents start 'bonding rituals' like eating ice-cream, chocolates, cakes and such desserts after meals. Worse, they allow meals to be eaten in front of the television, which results in children wanting to extend leisure time by way of mindless eating.

Urbanization-related intake behaviours that have been shown to promote obesity include frequent consumption of meals at fast food outlets, consumption of oversized portions at home and at restaurants, eating high calorie foods such as high-fat, low-fibre foods, and intake of sweetened beverages. These behaviours are cultivated environments where calorie-dense foods are abundant, affordable, available and easy to consume with minimal preparation. Hence, the trend is prevalent in urban cities across the country. Television viewing and other sedentary activities have also been related to childhood obesity. Unfortunately, this habit is growing exponentially in developing countries as well.

Parental failure to recognize childhood obesity is a major public health concern because parents regulate both what a child eats and their opportunities for physical activity. According to an article in *Pediatrics*, the official journal of the American Academy of Pediatrics, 'Parental perceptions of the child's weight status are a key part of many obesity intervention and prevention programmes. School measurement programmes in the UK and the US provide parents with feedback about their child's weight status. The cornerstone of such programmes rests on the assumption that parents will be better placed to address their child's weight when they perceive it accurately. Evidence of the effectiveness of these types of interventions is limited, and it is not clear whether altering parental perceptions of the child's weight status has an effect on the child's weight. Although accurate parental identification of child weight is an important step in challenging childhood obesity, an opposing view is that the stigma attached to the label of being 'overweight' may actually be more harmful than beneficial. Being overweight is a stigmatized condition and identifying oneself as overweight is stressful. It is associated with maladaptive coping responses that could lead to weight gain. For example, regardless of actual weight, adolescents who reported having been labelled as 'fat' by a family member or peer were more likely to become obese nearly a decade later,[13] as shown in Figure 2.1.[14]

Table 2: Perception of parents and children on influence of peer groups on children's eating behaviour

Healthy food behaviour (Eating Healthy Foods/ Learn Healthy food habits/ Intake Decreased)	1+	1+	2+
Unhealthy food behaviour (Intake increased/ Overeating/ Unhealthy Eating)	1+	2+	3+
Influence (not specified)	2+	2+	<1+
No Influence	2+	2+	1+

Note: In table 2, <1+ means 'Very few', 1+ meaning 'Some', 2+ meaning 'Approximately half', 3+ means 'Majority', 4+ meaning 'Most' and 5+ means 'Almost all'.

---

[13] Eric Robinson and Angeline R. Sutin, 'Parental perception of weight status and weight gain across childhood', https://www.ncbi.nlm.nih.gov/pmc/articles/PMC4845878/.

[14] http://inclentrust.org/inclen/wp-content/uploads/6_D2_Rakesh-Pillai_Thesis_03_Mar_18.pdf.

Given the economic constraints that force both parents to work; grandparents emerge as caregivers. They are usually indulgent and unmindful of their grandchild's size. They give in to the child's demands— be it a burger right after a traditional meal or a cola after evening play.

These are some uneasy social truths that we have to accept so that solutions can flow. Parents need not wait until their children are 50 per cent heavier than the ideal weight to seek a doctor's advice. The realization that their child is growing up as an obese individual should hit them sooner.

Physical activity is usually undervalued and prescribed as a ritual that is to be heard and forgotten about but resorted to in dire situations. Activity must be measured and parents should bond with their children and limit technology/screen time. Of course, parents alone cannot be blamed. Our governments have not focused on providing open spaces for play. Without open spaces, it is difficult to motivate children to take up physical activity. Moreover, parents are worried about their child's safety if they play on roads.

Overweight children don't like to exercise and it is not advisable to use the gym in the first fifteen years of life. Therefore, parents have to coax their child to take up some indoor game, such as badminton or table tennis. But, at the same time, they cannot push their child to play long hours; their child won't be competing in these sports but only playing for fun (and to burn some calories).

Lack of physical activity is the biggest bane of this generation, resulting in Size XL becoming an unhappy reality.

Chapter 3

No Child Is Fat Alone

In several Indian homes, especially in joint families or traditional households, the obesity juggernaut starts rolling when the child is an infant. Have you ever seen a child being fed by their mother in conventional Bollywood movies? We see no concept of satiety here as the mother piles food on the child's plate. Funny, right? We come from a land where an imposing potbelly is perceived as a symbol of accumulated power and not fat.

That is how we usually try to portray an Indian parent—we assume one should be like Devi Annapoorna, always cooking and feeding without understanding the concept of 'no', 'enough' or 'Please, I am full'. How can we blame 'mothers' love' when that alone is not the reason for today's obesogenic environment where the child is raised?

They stuff their toddlers with lovingly prepared mashed bananas, dal water or baby formula until they appear to gag. Only the loud protests of the child can get a mother to stop feeding them. The idea is to feed the child till they reach retching point. This method is flawed since it fills the child's stomach beyond capacity. Over the years, as the child is fed beyond this capacity, their stomach becomes accustomed to being stretched and expanded. This means that they will need more food to achieve satiety, as their stomach is now considerably bigger. What is the end result? Generation XL.

Have you ever tried understanding the riddle of rising obesity in the current generation as compared to our grandfathers and ancestors before them? Most of us have heard sermons exalting previous generations for their relatively active lifestyle, while emphasizing the growing inactiveness of Generation Z. Despite sounding clichéd, it is the truth. Our parents likely ate the same amount of food (more organic in nature with copious sweets and ghee and no concept of vegan, ketogenic or similar diets). Can you believe we are actually feeding on an entirely new nutritional industry today?

The word 'exercise' is so clichéd that today, we cannot think beyond yoga mats, treadmills and jogging parks.

But we will equivocally agree that our parents and grandparents engaged in ample exercise that helped them metabolize all the food they consumed which, to us, seem like calorific nightmares given our current lifestyles.

In an age where obesity is a global epidemic, this food is instead stored as fat (We are a nation that still strongly believes in debit than credit). Thus, it is imperative that we reconsider this native idea of the plump, healthy baby to prevent future generations from suffering for their increasingly sedentary lifestyles.

Whenever I receive patients struggling with their weight, I conduct a detailed analysis of their lifestyle, eating patterns and genetic history. Usually, we find a social or an emotional cause for the excessive weight gain. These often point to some lifestyle-related issue that is fuelling their obesity. Because the case with children is often more complex, I often break the scenario down for them and their parents. A child's family is often either unwittingly contributing to, or supporting the unhealthy behaviour patterns of their child.

Scientific literature backs up this claim. It suggests that the high prevalence of obesity and physical inactivity is caused by numerous individual, social and environmental factors. While no single factor is the primary cause, it is the congregation of many factors that have perpetuated the rise of overweight children and subsequent conditions. The entanglement of social, environmental and behavioural factors presents a complex challenge when identifying strategies aimed at addressing this problem. A key concept linked to obesity in children is that of obesogenic environments. Let us understand what they are.

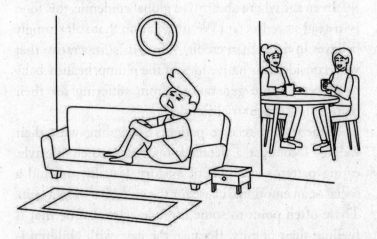

The doctor said he needed more activity, so I hid the TV remote thrice this week.

Obesogenic Environments

Let us go through the routine of a teenager from Mumbai, which is where most of my patients hail from. They are exposed to three different environments: one at school, another at home and the third depends on socio-economic status and preferences. It is one where the child spends time with friends, playing sports, video games, watching television, etc. A child spends approximately one-third of the day in each of these environments on a daily basis. Consequently, the people that populate these surroundings are bound to have some influence on the eating patterns of the child, especially since at least two, if not all three, involve eating. A child eats their tiffin, or buys food from the canteen in school, consumes regular meals at home, and, depending on the age of the child, might also snack with friends. School, home and the social environment also dictate the extent of physical exertion. This, along with the amount of time they spend in these environments, is a huge determinant of the child's BMI. Given the stubbornness of obesity as a disease, childhood habits and the resulting weight can be a lifelong problem that the child will have to contend with. The specific roles played by these environments are elaborated upon subsequently.

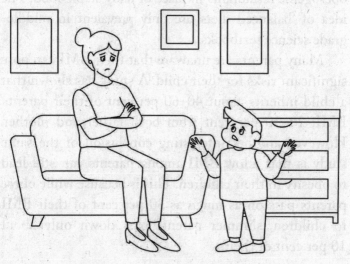

But I do exercise, Mom. I surf the Internet.

Environment 1 (home)

As the beginning of this chapter stated, the obesity epidemic usually begins at home. The kind of food a parent feeds their children can influence their diet as adults. For example, if as adults you love a full-course meal topped with sweets, you are passing on similar eating habits to your children without the awareness that what we eat makes up much of our physical self.

This is usually observed in joint or traditional families, where each and everything is a cause of celebration, and starts and ends with food. Its antithesis is evident in nuclear cosmopolitan families where it is rare to cook and normal to order food from outside. To keep up with Facebook and Instagram, we usually resort to branded, obesogenic restaurants in place of daily staple food. The idea of 'balanced diets' are only prevalent in middle-grade science textbooks.

Many parents are unaware that their BMI can pose significant risks for their child. A study has shown that a child inherits about 40–60 per cent of their parents' BMI, 20–30 per cent from both father and mother. However, another interesting conclusion of the same study is that a low BMI among parents can still lead to obesity in their children. This is because while obese parents pass on as much as 30 per cent of their BMI to children, slimmer parents pass down only about 10 per cent of theirs.

Besides their own weight, parents influence several variables that can exacerbate the risk of obesity in their progeny. Children can inherit genetic defects that make them prone to obesity. Though the percentage of children who are overweight due to a mutation is extraordinarily low, those who do have the condition need to be extra careful. Often, when parents have two children, one of whom is obese and one with normal weight, they feed them the same amount of food. While parents must consistently control and monitor their child's diet, considerable research has shown that improper restriction of meals worsens things, ending with an increase in the child's weight despite good intentions.

Parents misjudge their child's weight and fail to notice indicators of obesity at nascent stages when the disease can be controlled. They cannot comprehend the concepts of BMI, BMI percentile and BMI z-score. They rely on opinions from friends and family, which are misleading, since they do not have scientific or professional expertise. These opinions are also detrimental to the child's mental well-being and self-image.

The resulting confusion leads to them determining their child's weight by comparing with extreme cases seen in the media, or with the child's peers. They also rely on feedback from family members, who themselves might misjudge the child's weight. An easy remedy for this is scheduling regular check-ups with a doctor to ensure nothing is amiss. In the event of any issues, the doctor will be able to provide the requisite care that the child needs.

Comments regarding a child's weight are incredibly persistent in their memory and can be damaging for them in the long run. Girls who were told they were 'too fat' by or before age 10 were more likely to feel distressed about their weight, regardless of what their BMI actually is. They were also more likely to be obese than those who had not experienced unpleasant comments. The relation between a child's parents is another vital determinant of their weight. A child whose parents fight often is more likely to overeat due to stress.

Lastly, the educational level of parents is also correlated with childhood obesity. Parents with high education levels have often been shown to have slimmer children. This points to a viable solution that can potentially minimize the risk posed to a child's health. Spreading information and awareness regarding paediatric obesity can fight this epidemic, and institutions like the National Health Service (NHS) in the UK have recognized and implemented measures in line with this conclusion. This, along with regular visits to a doctor, can holistically improve a child's health, since it can help identify obesity at the earliest stage.

Likewise, having a health-conscious environment in a family where parents also aspire to be healthy and fit goes a long way to break the monotony of a sedentary lifestyle.

Environment 2 (school)

Schools are supposed to be bastions of education and knowledge. A school, however, is also a competitive environment, and as teens or pre-teens, children are constantly comparing themselves to peers. This can extend well beyond academics. Children can casually interact with their friends without fearing punishment from their teachers during recess, or during physical activity classes. But competition doesn't take a backseat even during these times. We all remember feeling jealous of that one friend who always brought delicacies to school while staring at our fruit-filled tiffins. Many were also given money by their working moms to eat from the canteen. Some of our healthier friends brought multiple tiffins with different foods. These have a profound influence on our own eating habits and food preferences. Resisting the temptation of canteen food can be difficult for adults, let alone children. Even if the canteen serves healthy food, there can be a plethora of street food options available close to schools. While junk food is convenient for working parents and appealing to children in school, parents must make time to ensure that their child is eating healthy. Children themselves might be incredibly persistent in their desire to eat this incredibly appetizing, but ultimately harmful food, and parents often do not have the patience to argue and remain firm on their stand. While it is a mentally draining exercise, the benefits make it a worthwhile endeavour.

Eating healthy and exercising go hand-in-hand in every area of life, and the same is true for schools. The World Health Organization (WHO) has recommended that all children between 5–17 years of age must do an hour of intensive exercise on a daily basis. Most schools in Mumbai, which is also my city of practice, have a single physical exercise (PE) session once a week. And that single session is not enough to counter the junk consumed by children. This trend is not restricted to India. Globally, around 80 per cent of all adolescents were insufficiently physically active. Countries like the UK, the US and Canada, have implemented several policies to ensure availability of safe and healthy food in schools. These include breakfast and lunch programmes that provide nutritionally balanced food at low costs, or even for free. In addition to this, public policy must mandate guidelines on PE sessions in schools. This will ensure that the training is not taken lightly, since the Indian government does not mandate requirements for PE training. It will also encourage schools to hire trained professionals who can guide children proficiently. Obese kids become a target for bullies. Even seemingly good-natured remarks can cause significant damage to one's self-esteem. This can lead to absenteeism and emotional stress that can cause overeating, depression and a general distraction from learning and growing as an individual. Though schools are only part of the problem, the mentioned solutions can make life easier for many students struggling with the disease.

Schools today are in a rush to garner fame and glory. For academic pursuits, sports periods are neglected or overlaid with academic classes. Such actions send out wrong messages to students as well as parents, denoting physical activity secondary to academics.

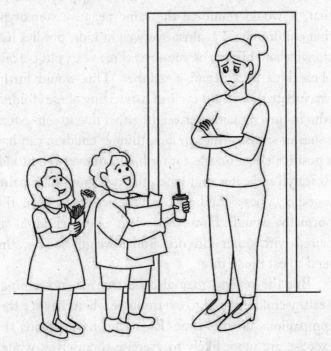

Can Johnny come out to eat?

Environment 3 (recreational time)

Besides parents and classmates, a child's choice of friends outside these two spheres is the third large determinant of paediatric obesity. There may be some overlap between friends who are classmates and those in the play area, but significant differences can exist too. This variable is perhaps the hardest to control, since one can't simply stop being friends with another just for being overweight. Even if one could hypothetically do that, it would reinforce the same negative stereotypes that children hold against overweight kids. Studies have shown that children as young as three years old perceive obese kids in a negative manner. This would further exacerbate the vicious cycle of ostracizing obese children, who in turn remain overweight either due to self-esteem issues or stress eating. In fact, thinner children can have a positive effect on the eating habits of overweight kids. Research indicates that when the two groups are paired together, obese children consume less food than they normally would. However, when obese children are paired with other kids in similar weight ranges, they tend to eat much more.

But the reverse may also be true when seemingly healthy children tend to overindulge when they see their companions do the same. Kids who have friends that exercise are more likely to exercise themselves, while a group of friends that prefer the sofa over playing outside will similarly influence a child to do the same. What's alarming is that obese children aren't just lazier than slimmer kids, but that they perceive exercise as an activity more negatively than kids with a lower BMI. This can determine one's attitude towards physical activities for a lifetime. It is hard to determine whether the positive influences outweigh the negatives, but at least one study suggests that the negative impact is stronger. Regardless of the truth, it is indisputable that friends do influence one another.

The key here seems to be to have more friends. Enrolling children into physically intensive activities, such as sports, self-defence, etc., can help them appreciate the benefits of exercise from an early age. Larger social groups can have a positive effect on everyone involved if most children in the group have healthy habits. Positive interactions with friends and peers are thought to have a significant impact on obesity. Being ostracized can have severe consequences for obese children. The pain of being excluded has been shown to be similar to physical pain. It disrupts their ability to self-regulate and to rely on their own judgments. Furthermore, children have a need for approval from their friends. Being ostracized can preoccupy these kids with finding a coping mechanism for their distress. For children, food is an easily accessible 'comfort', available to cope with distress.

The effect of peers on eating habits and its correlation to obesity risk is perhaps the most understudied of the three environments. As such, further research is needed to make more accurate and individual-specific judgments on solutions for their unique issues. However, based on the available information, maximizing the number of friends and engagements can counter the negative aspects of a social network on overcoming obesity.

Media and Our Relationship with Food

Media shapes our perception of food in subtle ways. Regardless of how active a child is, it is likely that at the end of the day, they spend hours in front of a television, iPad or a smartphone for entertainment. Through these gadgets, marketing and advertising play a particularly significant role in shaping norms and practices, especially for children. As per a report in the *International Journal of Behavioural Nutrition and Physical Activity*, 'Children view between 20,000 and 40,000 commercials per year, and food accounts for over 50 per cent of all ads targeting children. Children view an average of one food ad in every five minutes of TV viewing time.'[15] Food advertising is also targeted towards youngsters, since they are potentially lifelong customers. Because of the enormity of corporate interests in the promotion of unhealthy foods,

---

[15] Mary Story and Simone French, 'Food advertising and marketing directed at children and adolescents in the US', https://www.ncbi.nlm.nih.gov/pmc/articles/PMC416565/.

excessive eating and physical inactivity, changes are needed in policies that impact the food and physical activity environment. In California and in other states in the US, new statewide and local policies have been adopted to eliminate the sale of sodas and junk food from school campuses. Taxes have also been imposed to discourage the purchase of soda. Policies cannot rein in the freedom of corporations to advertise food to kids, but they can take measures to regulate the food itself, so that even if children are tempted to reach for a burger, they have some incentive not to. If the food is regulated, children might get something that is healthier to consume.

An obvious solution here is to reduce the children's screen time to no more than three hours a day. Studies show that among very young kids, those who watched more than three hours of television were 50 per cent more likely to be obese compared to those who didn't watch as much TV. It is also important to keep the child's screen time from increasing too much over a period, since many kids tend to consume high calorific food while watching television. Besides the statistics, reducing screen time makes sense because the more time a child spends with electronic gadgets, the lesser time they spend playing outside. Not only does this reduce the exposure to advertisements, but also ensures better sleep quality. Children who watch more television are known to have more sleep disturbances, which has been cited as a prominent cause of unhealthy eating habits. Thus, a TV in the child's bedroom is one thing all parents should avoid. It is of utmost importance to find the right balance for each individual between an optimal level of exercise and screen time, but the influence of media stretches far beyond merely television.

Hoardings, billboards and print or digital advertising showcase unrealistic beauty standards. Similar stereotypes are perpetuated by magazines and beauty pageants. They have the same pernicious effect, especially on girls, who are pressurized to adhere to certain standards from an early age. Lastly, social media also represents a flawed idea of beauty and fitness. Photo editing softwares alter images to blur out blemishes and marks on the face, and distort proportions to make individuals appear slimmer. Some applications also morph imagery to create bigger eyes, higher cheekbones and mutate out the natural skin colour, pigments, lines and other characteristics. While the 'beauty' of such photos is debatable, it does propagate a fake idea of 'good skin' and bodily proportions. This creates a false perception in the masses who believe the fake pictures. Such unbelievably good skin, hair and body are impossible to attain without the doctor's knife and a host of photo editing tools. Despite the intuitive conclusion that such imagery would encourage children to lose weight, they promote unrealistic body and beauty standards. The failure to achieve them despite long-term efforts can dishearten the child and they may fall back to their old habits and gain more weight.

Public Health Policy

Historically, methods to reduce obesity have focused on traditional medical models of behaviour modification, or treatment such as medicines, surgery, etc. In order to address health disparities and the larger social and environmental factors that influence them, obesity prevention efforts must include public policy as part of the solution. Some potential issues that are being considered as targets for action or mobilization include:

1. Competitive foods in schools
2. Physical Education in schools
3. Super-sized portions
4. Access for walking and bicycling
5. Advertising and promotion of unhealthy foods to children
6. Lack of institutional support for breastfeeding
7. Soda and sweetened beverages

Given the highly ethical nature of the debate, there are some issues with using public policy as a vehicle to combat obesity. These issues also inhibit the formation of any strong consumer-based movement that pushes for extensive legislation. Food companies make a wide range of products, some of which are healthy and some that are unhealthy. The food industry serves an important function by producing foods for mass consumption in the least amount of time possible. Policy levers affecting the nature of food products are related to agricultural subsidies, trade agreements, environmental policies, food labelling, demand and supply, etc. The health of the consumer is not considered since they are free to not purchase products and other food related items. This is probably why efforts to get the Federal Trade Commission (FTC)[16] to adopt measures that limit the amount of unhealthy foods marketed towards children have failed miserably. Children younger than a certain age do not usually have the agency to purchase products at the supermarket, and the responsibility of healthy eating choices falls on the parents. Yet, misleading advertisements can be disputed through legal discourse, but companies with competent firms fighting their court cases are seldom affected by such petitions or legal action.

Even in cases where policy measures have been adopted in an effort to curb obesity, some of the results have been highly disappointing. This has especially been the case with soda taxes. Sodas (sweetened beverages) may be easily targeted as they have zero nutritive value

---

[16] The FTC is a US federal agency that enforces antitrust laws and protects consumers.

and are positioned as a children's beverage. However, Hungary, Mexico, France and several states in the US have seen the policy fail when it comes to reducing obesity. To cite an example, when the residents of Philadelphia were faced with an increase in tax on soda, they reacted by shifting all their grocery purchases to stores beyond state borders. This caused financial losses worth millions for small and large businesses in the state, while those in neighbouring states thrived. The tax has resulted in such dire consequences that reports have warned of an incoming 'food desert' where nutritious food will be entirely unavailable in disadvantaged neighbourhoods, since many local markets have been forced to shut down. This indicates that even if public policy responds to the needs of a community, the community too must respond to these changes and adjust lifestyles accordingly.

Weight management is universally perceived as a matter of individual choice and discipline. Excessive weight is commonly associated with self-indulgence and gluttony. The public has been slow to link the obesity epidemic with an environment that is promoting unhealthy eating along with physical inactivity. While progress has been made in identifying unhealthy foods and food environments, particularly in schools, the need to change these environments through policy is urgent. Resources invested in the promotion of weight loss strategies through diet, pharmaceuticals and surgery as a quick fix, shift the focus away from prevention that begins at a young age. Reframing these issues in a way that builds public support for broader policy solutions to enable the public to implement these changes is crucial. It is also important to come up with comprehensive policies that look beyond isolated products such as soda, instant noodles or chips alone, since cutting out one unhealthy item does not guarantee weight loss. Lastly, education and awareness programmes can have a transformative impact on parents who are generally ill-equipped to deal with an obese child. As has been mentioned, many parents are confused by concepts like BMI owing to lack of knowledge.

Many children from low-income families live in communities with few resources and detrimental social and environmental factors (pervasive fast food outlets, little access to healthy food, no safe play and physical activity areas) that lead to childhood obesity and Type 2 diabetes. Intervening by changing the physical environment is the most successful and cost-effective prevention strategy for these children.

Obesity prevention efforts require numerous points of intervention, such as food security and food assistance programmes, schools and childcare settings, urban planning, public recreational facilities and healthcare settings. A focus on changing the food and physical activity environment helps build a strong social movement. We are up against a formidable industry, one with vast resources, far larger than anything we could bring to bear on this issue. We need a strong consumer-based movement to begin changing social norms around the causes and solutions for the challenges of overweight and obesity. We also need to raise awareness about obesity prevention and focus strategies on changing food and physical activity environments to enable everyone, especially those with the fewest resources, to practice healthy habits.

Part 2

Chapter 4

How Can I Help?

When a family seeks help for their obese child, doctors commonly begin with a conservative plan that focuses on diet. Alongside counselling, the family is advised on diet plans and daily calorific intake. For some children, the doctor may advise an exercise programme coupled with behavioural change, a nutritionist and a mental health professional's expertise along with the doctor's guidance.

It cannot be reiterated enough that obese children are at a high risk of suffering from chronic diseases later in life. They are more likely to develop diabetes, heart problems, osteoarthritis as well as a plethora of psychosocial problems, such as anxiety or depression. Medical research links obesity to stroke and cancer as well.

Experts have been talking about the obesity epidemic among children for years now. Their fears ring true every time one sees a gathering of children where at least a third of them are overweight. This is increasingly true not only of India's urban hubs, but even smaller cities and towns. The obesity epidemic among adults in India is estimated to be such that 30 to 65 per cent of adults are overweight, obese or have abdominal obesity. Among children, it is estimated that 20 to 30 per cent of children below 18 years of age are obese.

Studies carried out in the US suggest that half to three-quarters of obese children and teenagers will become obese adults.

We seem to know the problem: weight gain among children and teenagers who are not only physically inactive but also consume more calories than previous generations. But the solution to this problem is not as clearly spelt out. This could be partly attributed to the fact that obesity is still a nascent science as compared to, perhaps, infectious diseases. It was only in 2013 that the American Medical Association (AMA) recognized obesity as a disease. In fact, till 2008, an AMA team had held that obesity is a serious and complex condition that leads to numerous physical, emotional and social problems.

The medical community has, over the years, worked out a checklist to help families who are fraught with their child's obesity. It involves diet modification and family intervention where the family and child mend their food habits to maintain optimum weight. Counselling and behaviour therapy is known to help immensely. When these lifestyle modifications don't work, the treatment has to be taken to the next level i.e., medicines. If they fail too, surgery becomes the final choice. Studies suggest that lifestyle modification, along with parental support, works best for most children. But it must be questioned whether this practice would be too slow to be adequately helpful for the child.

Obesity among children isn't simple. It is not only a result of over-eating and not engaging in physical activity. Many factors are at play here: the child's genes, hormonal cycles that dictate metabolism, sleep cycles, their family's socio-economic status and lifestyle choices. These come down to everyday choices like travelling by automobiles, not climbing the stairs because they live on the twenty-sixth floor, etc. These seemingly unconscious choices all contribute to obesity among children.

Years ago, I conducted a survey on the weight and BMI of children attending a school that was located in a lower middle-class locality in Mumbai. They lived in simple settlements; didn't pursue many extra classes or own gizmos that would keep them glued to sofas. It implied that most children would be of appropriate weight.

My happiness was short-lived because during a subsequent interview linked to the study, the students confessed that they had a high affinity for junk food, such as pastries and pizzas. The seemingly healthy bunch was clearly unhealthy, and at a high risk of gaining weight in the future.

Should they be blamed for preferring junk food and thereby exposing themselves to a high risk of obesity? The reply cannot be a straight 'yes' or 'no'. The answer, painful though it may be for parents to hear, is what renowned American talk show host Oprah Winfrey once said, 'No child is fat alone.'

In the next three chapters, I suggest three methods to combat obesity.

Step 1 is the most essential component—Calorie Talk—where details and awareness about the nutrition and diet are illustrated. Often, we think that a dietician or nutritionist deprives and curtails our food choices. On the contrary, a nutrition-based approach makes us aware of the varied choices available at hand and how those foods enrich our body. It is very difficult to refuse children with palatable food options or make them follow a diet plan. Moreover, it is hard to impress upon them the consciousness of nutritious eating if they have not understood it from their early years. Often, their relationship with food is heavily dictated by peers as well as the media. In this section, with the help of charts based on food groups and interesting DIY meal plans, we intend to create a habit of 'eating right'. These charts are for both kitchen tac boards and school canteens. Also, for parents incessantly planning their weekly or monthly menus, we have created some family food planners and shopping checklists. For those parents who are ushering their children on the difficult road of weight loss, key pointers for diet planning have been suggested. This section deepens one's understanding on what kind of food combinations to consume for various age groups and weight groups. Some interesting recipes accompany these charts and checklists. Drafted along with nutritionist Indrayani Pawar, we hope the section is a comprehensive guide. Remember, diet forms the most essential component of a weight loss programme.

Step 2 is a corollary to the first step—a lifestyle modification. I advise the entire family to adopt this. It not only provides peer support to the child, but promotes an overall healthy attitude in the family that is sustainable. If diet maximizes weight loss, exercise tones the muscles and body and increases flexibility, strength and mobility.

Step 3 illustrates the physical activities and exercises that are essential accomplices for your child to maintain optimum health. It is important to understand that rigorous exercises at gyms are meant for adults but are not recommended for children due to multiple reasons. Their bones are still developing, so rigorous physical activity can be more harmful than useful. Hence, it is necessary to offer age-appropriate advice that is creative and engaging. For example, taking the child to a park or on playdates, and restricting their time with online devices, is an unpleasant but necessary parenting challenge.

Clearly, working out the appropriate treatment option is complex and, at times, a difficult process. If diet or exercise doesn't work, the next step is usually introduction of cognitive behaviour therapy to help the child combat obesity. This is what the chapter on 'Step 4' briefly covers. The use of medicines to treat childhood obesity is not encouraged owing to their side effects. In recent years, bariatric surgery for children, especially teenagers, has emerged as an option so that their health doesn't suffer further. However, I cannot stress enough about the personal commitment and the collaborative effort that the family must undertake as a unit to create positive change in the child's health. You can use the next section of the book to underline, make notes, tear away, etc.—the essential steps that are outlined for a healthy life and generation ahead.

Calorie Awareness

In the journey of weight loss, it is imperative to note that diet is more crucial than exercise. Exercises will help tone muscles but diets enable weight loss. Exercises can only supplement what a stringent diet can achieve. Hence, a dietician must ensure that the patient consumes adequate nutrition without eating in excess.

I would say that the dietician has to work like a mathematician to chart out the perfect meal course for an obese child. More importantly, they need to consider the fact that diet food cannot be tasteless nor include alien or unpalatable fare.

Day-to-day monitoring is essential for the dietician to check and make sure that weight lost is fat loss and not muscle loss. The core of the process is that diets should be tailored, controlled and, most importantly, people should understand that it is a gradual process. There are no shortcuts. Losing and maintaining weight alongside a healthy diet is not like medication or a short-term undertaking that ends once the child achieves their ideal weight. It is a lifestyle choice and must be adopted in a manner that can be sustained lifelong. While diets can jumpstart weight loss, we are looking at gradual but effective changes, a shift in mindset and actions that are upheld for life.

Alongside diet, children should be made aware of the harms of junk food and implications of obesity. This awareness is not merely about nutritional values but also about developing healthy relationships with food. Food is often used as a bribe or for positive reinforcement among children. Food must be perceived as nourishment with the occasional mindful indulgence in chips, chocolates and cola. The difference between 'eating for pleasure' and 'eating for nutrition' has to be defined and adhered to.

They should be made aware that although the diet may seem difficult and unpalatable initially, it will save them from many health issues in the future.

Of course, it is not possible for a person, especially a child, to maintain a diet for long durations. I have noticed that people tend to quit once they lose the first five kilos. This happens when the diet is too stringent or the person feels that they can ease restrictions after they achieve initial success.

What they fail to realize is that they could gain seven kilos within a few weeks or months after stopping the diet. This is because an obese person's stomach has become accustomed to stretch a lot for years and a few months of dieting and willpower may not be enough to stop this conditioned behaviour.

Understanding how one became overweight in the first place is an important step towards breaking the cycle. Most cases of childhood obesity are caused by excessive eating and a lack of exercise. Children need enough food to support healthy growth and development. But when they consume more calories than they burn throughout the day, the result is weight gain.

So, I have broken down the discussion about nutrition into these seven essential conversations:

1. Busting and clearing **myths and facts** (and a bonus quiz!)
2. Tips about eating **the right way**
3. Finally, the **calorie talk**
   - Dr Borude's food charts
   - Age-appropriate nutrition (energy chart)
4. Then we have a **star food chart** with age-appropriate food groups mentioned. This is something I would recommend that you tear away and paste up on your kitchen tac boards or secure on the fridge with magnets.

5. How can we not include some **culinary lessons** based on the above food chart that can be tried by all at home, for weekend cooking parties or even the everyday lunch box?
6. Finally, **fuel up** with lunch box ideas, food planners and shopping lists.

So, let's begin by testing your smarts about nutrition or food.

 TEST YOUR SMARTS!

Adolescents have special nutrition needs, different from other people.

True | False

It's best to eat three meals a day. No snacking!

True | False

Only adults need to worry about getting enough calcium.

True | False

You don't have to completely give up burgers, fries, ice cream and all that, if you want to eat healthy.

True | False

It is okay to eat whatever you want as long as you exercise.

True | False

Eliminating foods like carbohydrates, fat and sugar will make you skinny.

True | False

Fast food is always fattening.

True | False

Thin people are healthier than obese people.

True | False

Eating at night makes you fat.

True | False

Substitutes like aspartame for sugar, margarine for butter, cauliflower rice in place of regular rice are healthier.

True | False

Multiple small meals throughout the day are better than three huge meals.

True | False

Low-fat, fat-free and sugar-free foods have fewer calories.

True | False

Certain foods like cabbage soup and cucumber sticks help you lose weight.

True | False

Myths and Facts about Weight Problems and Obesity in Children

Myth 1: Childhood obesity is genetic, so there's nothing you can do about it.

Fact: While a person's genes do influence their weight, they are only one small part of the equation. Although some children are more prone to gaining weight than others, that doesn't mean that they are destined for weight problems. Most kids can maintain a healthy weight if they eat right and exercise.

Myth 2: Children who are obese or overweight should be put on a diet.

Fact: Unless directed by your child's doctor or otherwise, the treatment for childhood obesity is not weight loss. The goal should be to slow down or stop weight gain, allowing your child to grow into their ideal weight.

Myth 3: It's just baby fat. Children will outgrow the weight.

Fact: Childhood obesity doesn't always lead to obesity in adulthood, but it does raise the risks dramatically. The majority of children who are overweight at any time during preschool or elementary school are still overweight as they enter their teens. Most kids do not outgrow the problem.

The Right Way

So how do we get it right? Let's begin by making healthier food choices

While you may need to make major changes to your family's eating habits, changing everything all at once often leads to cheating or giving up. Instead, start by taking small, gradual steps towards healthy eating. Changes should be made in a gradual fashion rather than drastically overhauling eating habits. If the family is accustomed to desserts after meals, one can swap a fruit-based cake or pudding in place of ice cream or deep-fried sweets. Parents can then move on to reducing dessert quantities or meal portions to balance the calories consumed in the dessert. Similarly, if children tend to snack in front of the television, parents can offer fruit or snacks like 'kurmura' (puffed rice), seeds, etc. Add a salad to dinner every night or swap French fries for baked potatoes and later, baked potatoes with baked vegetables. The key is slow but steady progression into eating healthy. As these small changes become a matter of habit, you can continue to add more healthy choices.

A Visual Treat

There is always a way to create interesting patterns for children. One such way is to **eat the rainbow.** The diet can be designed to include red (beets, tomatoes), orange (carrots, squash), yellow (potatoes, bananas), green (lettuce, broccoli) and so on—just like eating a rainbow. Consumption of a wide variety of fruits and vegetables is encouraged but can be difficult to implement for children. But by gradually introducing healthier choices and sustaining them, the parent can create innovative recipes. Fruits can be frozen and served as popsicles; vegetables can be cut into strips and served to resemble pasta, etc. You can also explore recipes with your child and understand tastes that appeal to them and devise food accordingly.

You first eat with your eyes and this cannot be truer for children. Fussy eaters can be lured into eating a variety of food if presented invitingly, like a bowl of ice cream garnished with fruit or pasta made fun with colourful veggies like broccoli, purple cabbage, tomatoes, etc. You can also make a game out of identifying colours with younger kids.

For the older children, the parent must connect with aspirations that drive them. For someone, it could be excelling at sport, another may wish for enhanced concentration, better skin and hair or even 'aesthetic' food that they can photograph and share on social media. You can plug in food that fits with their desires, communicate the role of food and nutrition and embark on a joint effort to eat the rainbow.

Don't skip breakfast. Children who eat breakfast are less likely to be overweight or obese than those who skip the first meal of the day. It's important to focus on healthy choices like oatmeal, fresh fruit, whole grain cereal that is high in fibre and low in sugar and low-fat milk instead of sugary cereals, doughnuts or pastries. Breakfast can be the meal that the family eats together. You can enrol in an activity, sport, yoga class or equivalent with the entire family followed by a healthy and hearty breakfast. By building upon the previous cues of making healthier food choices and eating the rainbow, breakfast can be made a fun family affair before everyone sets off to work and study.

Look for hidden sugar. We know the obvious offenders that contain sugar. But reducing the amount of candy and desserts you and your child eat is only part of the battle. Sugar is hidden in foods like bread, canned soups, pasta sauce, pickles, frozen foods, low-fat meals, fast food and ketchup. The major culprits are health drinks and milk supplements, which are endorsed by leading athletes and celebrities. They mislead people into believing that milk alone does not contain enough nutrients and should be reinforced with powders for added nutrition. A major ingredient in these supplements is sugar. A popular cornflake brand implies that their packaged grub has more nutrition than almonds. Similarly, several health drinks that claim to have vitamin C are also laden with sugar. While advertisements do not directly make the above-mentioned claims, their ads lead people to absorb incorrect ideas related to these products.

The body gets the required amount of sugar from natural foods like fruits, milk and even some vegetables like potatoes, grains like rice, etc. Added sugar amounts to nothing but empty calories. And naturally available foods are abundant in nutrition but the multi-billion-dollar food industry would like us to believe otherwise. Instead of buying milk drinks or supplements to be added to milk, try creating healthier alternatives at home. Use cocoa powder and dates to recreate the lure of chocolate milk. Even the traditional masala milk with cardamom, saffron and dried fruits is packed with nutrition.

Check labels and opt for low sugar products. Choose and use fresh over frozen and frozen over canned. In short, choose the lesser evil to begin with and slowly but steadily, proceed towards eliminating sugar entirely.

Limit juice, soda and coffee drinks. Soft drinks are loaded with sugar. Shakes and packaged coffee drinks can be just as bad. Most juices offer little nutrition as the fibre is often discarded with the peel and pulp. Offer your child sparkling water with a twist of lime, fresh mint or a splash of fruit juice with pulp instead.

Don't ban sweets. While many kids consume too much sugar, a 'no sweets' rule invites cravings and overindulging when the chance arises. Instead, limit cookies, candies and baked goods that your child eats and introduce fruit-based snacks and desserts.

Schedule regular meal times. Children can get used to set routines. If your kids know they will only get food at certain times, they will be more likely to eat what they get when they get it.

Limit dining-out. If you must eat out, try to avoid fast food. Set restrictions firmly with respect to the occasions or number of times a month that fast food can be had. Make smarter food choices when eating at restaurants. Opt for steamed or baked items over fried—steamed dumplings, baked fish or chicken with vegetables, etc. You can order a side of salad without dressing, choose items with more vegetables than with refined ingredients such as vegetable pasta over mac-and-cheese and so on.

Don't go no fat; go good fat. Not all fats contribute to weight gain. Instead of trying to cut out fat from your child's diet, focus on replacing unhealthy fats with healthy fats.

Avoid trans fats that are dangerous to your child's health. Try to eliminate or cut back on commercially baked goods, packaged snacks, fried foods and anything with 'partially hydrogenated' oil in the ingredients, even if it claims to be trans fat free. It is impossible to avoid the lure of packaged cakes and chips that dot markets. A better idea would be to create these goodies at home. Let the child bear the responsibility of buying ingredients for cakes, chips or pasta to wean them away from shelves of instant noodles. Redirect their energy and inquisitiveness into healthier ingredients that can create similar but healthier options. Also, one must bear in mind that even though they may be made at home, cakes, pasta, chips, etc., do contain excessive calories and must be restricted.

Add more healthy fats that can help a child control blood sugar and avoid diabetes. Unsaturated or 'good' fats include nuts and seeds like peanuts, almonds and cashews. Eggs, avocados, olive oil, fatty fish, soy, tofu, flaxseed, etc. also consist of healthy fats. But they are also high in calories, so their consumption must be limited. Cooking fat like butter, ghee, coconut oil, mustard oil and unrefined oils are imperative to maintain health.

Choose saturated fat wisely. The United States Department of Agriculture (USDA) recommends limiting saturated fat to 10 per cent of your child's daily calories. Focus on the source of saturated fats consumed: a glass of whole milk or natural cheese rather than a hot dog, doughnut or pastry; grilled chicken or fish instead of fried chicken, etc.

Again, marketing and advertising play a huge role in the way we perceive fat. Some ads portray butter, ghee and traditional oils as 'harmful' and promote factory made margarine and substitutes in their place. But would you rather trust food from your ancestors' kitchens or one that is manufactured in a factory? Some brands also package ready-to-eat foods as 'trans fat free'. While the claim is true, do check for their calorific value versus nutritional value.

Be smart about snacks and sweet food. Your home is where your child most likely eats the majority of meals and snacks, so it is vital that your kitchen is stocked with healthy but interesting choices; khakhras, millet-based munchies, etc.

Keep snacks small. Don't turn snacks into a meal. Limit them to 100 to 150 calories. Dates, a bowl of chickpeas, sprouts chaat, home-made bhel and similar options can be considered.

Go for reduced sugar options. When buying foods such as syrups, jellies and sauces, opt for products labelled as with 'reduced sugar' or 'no added sugar'.

Focus on fruit. Keep a bowl of fruit out for your children to snack on. Offer fruit as a sweet treat—frozen juice bars, fruit smoothies, strawberries and a dollop of whipped cream; fresh fruit added to plain yogurt; or sliced apples with peanut butter. Better still, get children to choose the fruit of their liking and have them freeze it. Once frozen, they can serve and plate the dessert in creative ways. This is also a good way to get them to eat the rainbow.

Experiment with herbs and spices. Use sweet tasting herbs and spices such as mint, cinnamon, allspice, vanilla or nutmeg to add sweetness to food without the empty calories. For instance, sliced apples sprinkled with cinnamon are a great treat. You can also add dates for sweetness and bake them on a whole wheat crust to make your version of an apple pie.

Check the sugar content of your kid's cereal. There's a huge disparity in the amount of added sugar between different brands of cereals. Some cereals contain more than 50 per cent sugar by weight. Try mixing a low sugar, high-fibre cereal with your child's favourite sweetened cereal, or add fresh or dried fruit to oatmeal for a naturally sweet taste.

Watch portion sizes. There are strategies you can employ to retrain your family's appetites and avoid oversized servings when eating out. There are multiple ways you can ensure you are controlling your portion sizes.

Learn what a regular portion size looks like. The portion sizes that your family is used to eating may be equal to two or three true servings. To keep calories in check, use the hand as a measuring unit. For women, the size of their palm indicates the quantity of lean protein that they should consume; the fist the size of vegetables or salad, a cupped hand the portion of carbs like rice or starchy vegetables like potatoes. Finally, fat should only be a thumb-sized quantity. For men, double the quantities.

Read food labels. Information about serving size and calories can be found on the backs of packaging. You may be surprised at how small the recommended portions are or how many calories are in the dish. Most foods that are created with children as their target consumers are often high in sugar. Check for salt content, preservatives, food colour, etc. Most importantly, check the nutrition labels versus the calories they contain.

Use smaller dishes. The portions will look bigger and you'll eat less when you use small bowls or plates.

Dish up in the kitchen. To reduce second and third helpings, serve food on individual plates instead of putting the serving dishes on the table.

Divide food from large packages into smaller containers. The larger the package, the more people tend to eat without realizing it.

Cut up high-calorie treats, such as cheese, pizza, or chocolate, into smaller pieces and offer your child fewer pieces.

Downsize orders. When eating out, share an entrée with your child or just order an appetizer instead. Order half-portions or medium sizes instead of a large serving. Buffets can be avoided by visiting places that offer single serve options. Avoid the temptation to over order.

Sugary Drinks and Health

As per a report by the Harvard T. Chan School of Public health 'When it comes to ranking beverages best for our health, sugary drinks fall at the bottom of the list because they package calories and virtually zero nutrients. People who drink sugary beverages do not feel as full in comparison to if they had eaten the same calories from solid food. Research also indicates that they also don't compensate for the high caloric content of these beverages by eating less food. In fact, these drinks accompany meals. The average can of sugar-sweetened soda or fruit punch provides about 150 calories, almost all of them from added sugar. If you were to drink just one of these sugary drinks every day, and not cut back on calories elsewhere, you could gain up to five pounds in a year. Beyond weight gain, routinely drinking these sugar-loaded beverages can increase the risk of Type 2 diabetes, heart disease and other chronic diseases. Furthermore, higher consumption of sugary beverages has been linked with an increased risk of premature death.'[17]

---

[17] 'Sugary drinks', https://www.hsph.harvard.edu/nutritionsource/healthy-drinks/sugary-drinks/.

Cut back on sugary drinks. When it comes to our health, it's clear that sugary drinks should be avoided. There is a range of healthier beverages that can be consumed in their place, with water being the top option.

Of course, if your child is a frequent soda drinker, this is easier said than done. If it's the carbonation they like, give sparkling water a try. If the taste is too bland, try a naturally flavoured sparkling water. If that's still too much of a jump, add a splash of juice, sliced citrus or even some fresh herbs. You can do this with home brewed tea as well, like sparkling iced tea with lemon, cucumber and mint. You can keep flavoured water at home to minimize cravings. Try adding mint leaves and cucumber with lime; boil water with cinnamon for a sweetish flavour, etc.

What about 'diet' sodas or other drinks with low-calorie sweeteners?

According to another report by the Harvard T. Chan School of Public Health, 'Low-calorie sweeteners (LCS) are sweeteners that contain few to no calories but have a higher intensity of sweetness per gram than sweeteners with calories. These include artificial sweeteners, such as aspartame and sucralose, as well as extracts from plants like steviol glycosides and monk fruit.

Beverages containing LCS sometimes carry the label 'sugar-free' or 'diet'. The health effects of LCS are inconclusive with research showing mixed findings. A 2018 scientific advisory by the American Heart Association and American Diabetes Association noted that further research on the effects of LCS beverages on weight control, cardio-metabolic risk factors and risk of cardiovascular disease and other chronic diseases is needed. That said, they also note that for adults who are regular high consumers of sugary drinks, LCS beverages may be a useful temporary replacement strategy to reduce intake of sugary drinks.'[18]

Action Beyond the Individual Level

WARNING:
Drinking beverages
with added sugar(s)
contributes to obesity,
diabetes, and tooth decay.

[18] 'Low-calorie sweeteners', https://www.hsph.harvard.edu/nutritionsource/healthy-drinks/artificial-sweeteners/.

Sugar addiction is a serious issue. Reducing our preference for sweet beverages will require concerted action at several levels—from creative food scientists and marketers in the beverage industry, as well as from individual consumers and families, schools and worksites, and state and the federal government. We must work together towards an urgent cause: alleviating the cost and the burden of chronic diseases associated with obesity and diabetes epidemics in India. Fortunately, sugary drinks are a growing topic in policy discussions, both nationally and internationally.

The Calorie Talk

So, how many calories are you eating each day? How much fat? Getting enough vitamins, calcium, and iron? The Nutrition Facts label depicted in Figure 4.1 is the way you can tell. Here's a crash course.

The Nutrition Facts Label – Your Healthy Eating Tool

Nutrition Facts
Serving Size 1 cup (228g)
Servings Per Container 2

The top of the label tells you the size of one serving, and how many servings are in the package.
What matters here? Check the size of a serving. Is the portion you choose actually two, three or four servings? Then double, triple or quadruple the calories, vitamins, etc., you see on the rest of the label.

The Nutrition Facts Label – Your Healthy Eating Tool

Amount Per Serving

Calories 250   Calories from Fat 110

This section is about calories, and calories from fat.

What matters here? Regularly eating more calories than the body uses leads to having extra body weight to lug around. A rule of thumb for choosing foods—40 calories per serving means the food is low in calories, 100 calories/serving is moderate, and 400 or more is high.

	% Daily Value*
Total Fat 12g	18%
Saturated Fat 3g	15%
Trans Fat 3g	
Cholesterol 30mg	10%
Sodium 470mg	20%
Total Carbohydrate 31g	10%

Next come nutrients that we typically eat plenty (or too much!) of.

What matters here? A healthy eating style limits fat, cholesterol, and sodium (salt). The % Daily Value column is your 'cheat sheet.' If the column shows 5 per cent or less, the food is low in fat, or cholesterol, or sodium. If the column shows 20 per cent or more, the food is high in fat, cholesterol, or sodium.

The Nutrition Facts Label – Your Healthy Eating Tool

Dietary Fiber 0g	0%
Sugars 5g	
Protein 5g	
Vitamin A	4%
Vitamin C	2%
Calcium	20%
Iron	4%

This part lets you zero in on key nutrients we all need.

First is fibre. Then look below the black bar for vitamins, and two things that young people really need—calcium (for bones) and iron (for muscles and blood).

What matters here? Are the foods you eat delivering 100 per cent of the fibre, vitamins, calcium, and iron your body needs? Remember that foods without labels (like fresh fruits and veggies) count too!

* Percent Daily Values are based on a 2,000 calorie diet. Your Daily Values may be higher or lower depending on your calorie needs.

	Calories:	2,000	2,500
Total Fat	Less than	65g	80g
Sat Fat	Less than	20g	25g
Cholesterol	Less than	300mg	300mg
Sodium	Less than	2,400mg	2,400mg
Total Carbohydrate		300g	375g
Dietary Fiber		25g	30g

The Nutrition Facts Label – Your Healthy Eating Tool

Last, the footnote.

What matters here? The footnote provides a handy daily cheat sheet on how much you should be aiming for overall in terms of fat, cholesterol, sodium (salt), carbohydrates and fibre. This part of the label is the same on every food. (To make it easy for you, most kids aged 9–13 need about 2,000 calories per day.

FAQs about Your Diet (Must Read for the Child!)

 What is a healthy diet?

Eating a healthy diet means giving your body the type and amount of food and drinks that help it carry out its functions optimally and as a result, you look and feel your best. When you give your body what it needs (like vitamins, minerals and proteins), it uses the same to offer you much in return, like energy, powerful muscles and strong bones. The body functions like a high-performing machine that requires fuel to keep working efficiently. If the fuel is less, the machine (the body) will not work properly. You will suffer from weakness, lack of focus, hair loss and other such problems. On the other hand, if you add excessive fuel, it can damage the parts. In your body, this leads to excess weight, sluggishness and even problems in bowel movement. There are foods that fuel different functions, organs and systems in the body and it is important to eat all of them in the required quantities.

Q **What foods give my body what it needs for energy, muscles and all that?**

A It takes a variety of different foods. A healthy diet is made up mostly of whole grains, vegetables, fruits, low-fat dairy foods and smaller amounts of lean meats, fish and poultry (like chicken or turkey), pulses and beans. While we know that these foods are optimum for consumption and high on nutrients, it is essential to understand how these foods nourish the body. Whole grains like rice and wheat, millets like jowar, bajra and ragi and roots like potatoes, yams, colocasia, etc., are carbohydrates that provide energy.

Lean meats like fish, chicken, turkey, etc., and pulses and beans like chickpeas, rajma, tur, lobia and moong are sources of protein. Milk and milk products also contain proteins. Eggs are a nutritious and delicious source of protein too. Proteins are important to repair the wear and tear of the body. The body uses protein to make enzymes, hormones, muscle, cartilage, skin and bones. Basically, the body, bones, skin and flesh are all protein. Protein is what helps the body shed old skin cells and regenerate with new ones. Want great skin and hair? Eat your eggs and drink that dal! The occasional indulgence in red meat is okay, given that you eat in small quantities and perhaps only once a month. Else, stick to lean meats like fish, chicken and turkey.

So, you have energy from carbohydrates to move around, play, exercise and work. And proteins will build and repair your body. What else does your body need, you may wonder? Well, it needs to get rid of waste that is generated once the body absorbs nutrition from the food you eat. That's where fruits and vegetables enter the scene. Fruits and vegetables, like cabbage, cauliflower and spinach, and roots, like carrots, beets, etc., contain fibre that is necessary for bowel movement.

This puzzle seems complete since alongside energy and growth, excretion is also taken into account. But there is more to the body's functioning beyond growing and shedding excesses and the unwanted. You need to nourish the brain, care for vital organs, look after gut health and so on. You also need fat for energy, growth and many other functions.

Everybody needs plenty of water daily. Water is not only refreshing but your body needs it for its everyday functions from digesting food to circulating blood. Many foods, especially fruits and vegetables like cucumber, tomatoes, apples, oranges, etc. have high water content but it is important to drink water at regular intervals to keep the mind and body working just fine.

Q **How do I mix these food groups to make a complete meal?**

A The foods that we covered, carbohydrates, proteins and fruits and vegetables will take care of these functions. But it is important to understand how these food groups work together like cogs of a machine for overall performance and how to mix and match different groups for best results.

Fruits and vegetables are crucial because they pack in low calories but are very nutrient dense. Different fruits and vegetables contain minerals, vitamins, antioxidants and a host of other nutrients, which will become a huge matrix if every benefit is explained. The trick here is to eat the rainbow! It will add a variety of different tastes and textures onto your plate and you will get maximum benefits. Then it is important to eat meals in stipulated quantities; as per gender, age, height and physical activity levels.

Again, some sources of proteins are also rich in fat and carbohydrates. Like two large eggs (105 grams) have 13 grams protein and 11 grams fat.

Whole wheat flour is commonly eaten across the nation and it consists of 72.57 grams carbohydrates and 13.7 grams protein. Certain carbohydrate rich foods also contain vitamins, minerals and even calcium. Potatoes with skin have vitamin C, potassium, folate, etc.

but carbohydrates are a major constituent. While rice is mainly all carbohydrates, it does have some protein. Varieties like black rice have higher protein content than white rice and also have iron apart from being rich in antioxidants.

Some legumes pack in carbohydrates alongside protein. For instance, 100 grams rajma has 8.7 grams protein but 22.8 grams carbohydrate. On the other hand, 100 grams moong has 7.35 grams protein and 18.38 grams carbohydrates. It is interesting to note that wheat packs in more protein than dals, but one must remember that the former's major constituent is carbs. Similarly whole milk has proteins and carbohydrates in almost equal parts and also contains calcium. Paneer is made from milk when milk solids are separated from whey (by adding lemon or vinegar). Hence, 100 grams of paneer will have more protein than 100 grams of milk.

Q What are super foods? Is it important to eat super foods to maintain good health?

A Every once in a while, a certain fruit, vegetable, seed, nut, etc. makes waves on television and social media as the next big 'super food'. You may remember celebrities and public figures endorsing quinoa some years ago followed by kale recently. Avocados were all the rage once and currently, it is turmeric in the form of turmeric latte, golden milk and various other avatars.

Any whole food that is unprocessed, and is in its natural form without being treated with chemicals is a super food, in my opinion.

Any food, as long as it is locally grown, minimally processed and consumed whole, has 'super' benefits. For example, ripe bananas provide the body with vitamin B6, vitamin C, potassium, magnesium, fibre and other nutrients. Raw bananas, the green ones that are consumed cooked, also have benefits. Raw bananas have certain micro nutrients that diminish as they ripen, while ripe bananas have more antioxidants. Basically, bananas are great, economical and satiating. They do have 'super' qualities. But what happens when the same banana is converted into banana chips? There's oil that is re-used to fry the chips, a ton of salt and so, this super food becomes a health hazard if consumed in large quantities.

Similarly, let's take avocados. This source of healthy fats is great when eaten whole but if converted into a smoothie with added sugar, you are also consuming empty calories. Also, while avocados are being cultivated in India, the fruit is not native to our region. They are cultivated in select areas in the country. Avocados are surely gaining popularity and they may become as popular as zucchinis soon but currently, they are transported over great distances to reach the local market. Often, such produce is harvested raw and may be ripened with chemicals to extend their shelf life. This also extends their cost while their nutritional benefit may not be at par with avocados that are naturally available in their local habitat. While buying any food that is labelled as a super food by the media or by your favourite celebrity, do consider whether factors like transport, chemical processing and packaging diminish their 'super powers'. The best super foods are local and seasonal fruits and vegetables from markets near your home.

Q **So, if I want to eat a healthy diet, are there foods I have to skip completely?**

A No. There can be a place for everything.

Let's go back to the big picture. It's true, most of what you eat should be the foods that deliver what you need to look and feel your best. But if you're thinking that you haven't seen any mention of soda, corn chips, chocolate cake or pepperoni pizza yet, don't worry! These foods can fit into the puzzle. The goal is to track the four key elements:

1. Calories,
2. Fat,
3. Sugar,
4. Salts
5. Some foods (like sodas, potato chips, chocolate cake and pepperoni pizza) can pack a lot of calories, fat, sugar and/or salt. Getting too

much of these four key things can slow you down. And eating too much fat can also start clogging your arteries (blood vessels) with waxy goo. A treat once in a while is fine as long as you remember to eat within your calorific limit. The calorific limit is the number of calories a person needs to eat every day to meet their energy needs. Everyday activities like walking, breathing, digestion and even sleeping require energy. The calorie is the unit of measuring energy requirement, which has now become the generic term used to describe the amount of energy a food gives.

The calorific limit is determined by your age, gender, height and physical activity. If you eat more than what is stipulated, you gain excess weight. If you eat less than mandated, you will be tired and sluggish. And within the equation of balancing your calories, you must ensure that you eat foods that nourish your body in a balanced fashion. Remember we spoke about carbohydrates, proteins, minerals, fats and other food groups? And even the idea of eating minimally processed whole foods? Yes, you have to eat those foods in stipulated quantities. If you eat an overall healthy diet, the occasional chocolate, pizza or a handful of chips will not harm you. The key is balance.

Q **Is it okay to eat whatever I want as long as I am not exceeding my body's calorific limit?**

A No. Calorie counting is futile if you eat junk food like chips, samosas, pizzas and chocolates that have more empty calories and little nutrition. Your body, brain and organs will not get any nourishment and you will have deficiencies. It may lead to diseases also.

Q **What are the food items that lead to weight loss or can be eaten in unlimited quantities without an overload of calories?**

A You can eat fruits and vegetables with high water content. Cucumbers (96 per cent water), tomatoes (95 per cent water), mushrooms (92 per cent water), spinach (93 per cent water) and oranges (86 per cent water) are some fruits and vegetables that have high water content and low-calorific content. They are also nutritious, locally available and can be consumed with minimal cooking and processing. But, can you really sustain yourself on these foods? You also need rice, natural sugars and good fats for your well-being.

A large part of eating is also about satiety. We do want to eat healthy and be fitter, but we cannot deny that we also eat for emotional reasons. Food does impart a 'feel good' factor. If your food does not make you happy, you will not be able to sustain healthy eating habits for life. It is crucial that we accept that food is an important part of life; from nutrition to celebrations to emotional times. And once we realize this fact, it will be easier to be more conscious of our eating habits. You will know exactly what food has what effect on your body and mind. As a result, you will not be harsh on yourself for the occasional indulgence but will work towards burning the calories or consuming less in your next meal. Do not fall into either trap:

1. Sticking to your daily calorie goals but majorly consuming unhealthy foods.
2. Being excessively stringent and following a boring food routine.

Q **What about how MUCH food to eat?**

A Figure 4.2 has a list of the different kinds of foods people need and also gives you an idea as to how much you should consume each day. Kids who aren't very active need to eat less food than kids who are very active.

Nutrition labels talk about how many cups or any other unit of measurement make one 'serving' of that food. The labels show things like the fat, calories, and nutrition from vitamins that food gives you, if you eat one serving of it.

	9–13-year-olds		Measurement in
	Less Active	More Active	
Fruits	1 ½	↔ 2	cups
Veggies	2	↔ 3	cups
Grains (like whole grain bread, brown rice, popcorn)	3	↔ 7	ounces
Lean meat, poultry, fish, eggs, beans	5	↔ 6	ounces
Low-fat milk, yogurt, or cheese		3	cups
Fats or oils (like olive oil in salad dressing, oils in nuts)	5	↔ 6	teaspoons

Some things that may look like one serving are really much more. Next time you grab an individual-sized package of chips, cookies or crackers; check the label—these small-sized packages actually count as two or three servings, even though it would be easy to eat them all at once. Another good reason to be a label reader!

Q **Nutrition, Fruits and Vegetables, Calories, Fat . . . all over magazines, on the news, in school . . . Why is it such a big deal?**

A We need nutrition from foods and drinks to fuel our bodies. The kinds and amounts of food we give our bodies can directly affect how we look and feel. With the best (most nutritious) fuel, we're ready and able to do all the stuff we have to do, and all the stuff we want to do.

And, you're right—the world makes it a little complicated. However, it must be noted that fitness has been complicated and misrepresented. As many regular people struggle with weight, the media shows skinny women and muscular men as happier, healthier and better than others as they are more popular and successful. Watch any popular television show or movie; the lead actors and even the side actors will not have any flab, double chin or sagging skin. What they don't show you is the extent to which these images are digitally edited to flatten the stomachs and erase double chins. Even the skinniest person's stomach will show 'rolls and folds' when they sit. That's a normal body. Then we see these actors with their morphed bodies endorsing colas, chips, biscuits and other junk food during advertisements. And then there will be another commercial advertisement showcasing breakfast cereal, energy bars and magic pills that help you lose weight.

Even magazine and newspaper advertisements talk about food only in terms of weight loss or 'tasty' foods. While newspapers and magazines sometimes also talk about eating right through a column or special feature, they are overpowered by advertisements. Pick up any newspaper or magazine and look at the space that an advertisement occupies verses a regular column. The ads will be much more colourful and with bigger fonts to grab your attention. Ditto for ads on billboards atop buildings and on the roads!

So, while you know that you should be eating healthy, you are also constantly bombarded with images. Your brain starts processing ideas that are subtly embedded in these colourful, flashy ads: skinny equals successful and happy; food must either lead to weight loss or is eaten for pleasure; if I eat a certain cereal for breakfast, I will have a flat stomach; and so on.

There are occasions when food represents not only nutrition but also festivities, emotional eating etc. For example, when families cook huge meals to celebrate, or when one eats because they feel sad or others think grabbing fries instead of carrots is more convenient for the time being, etc.

Ready for some sanity? What is the bottom line? A healthy eating style is about fuelling your body in a healthy way to be your personal best.

The Star Food Chart:

AGE-APPROPRIATE FOOD GROUP

What a Child Should Eat

Indrayani Pawar

FOR CHILDREN
(Age group: 5–10 years)

Food group	Description	Reason	
Cereals	Whole wheat, ragi, jowar, oats, rice, makhana, rajgeera	Cereals give us carbohydrates, especially complex carbohydrates, with plenty of fibre and essential vitamins.	Kids of this group experience the increased burden of studies over a period of time. They need to eat enough complex carbohydrates to give them a constant supply of glucose for their ever- anxious brain.

Food group	Description	Reason	
			Ingredients like maida or refined wheat flour (read biscuits/bread/pizza/pasta) will give a short spurt of energy and, in fact, will leave your child drained.
Pulses	All dal and legumes (especially sprouted)	Proteins are the main building blocks and are required in good amounts at this age. Once sprouted, pulses are also an enriched source of vitamins and minerals.	Fussy eaters and vegetarians, especially, need to include this food group, to help body growth and to maintain wear and tear of tissues.

Food group	Description	Reason	
Vegetables	All green leafy vegetables, beans and gourd vegetables	Vegetables are power packed with all the essential vitamins and minerals required to aid proper growth at this age.	The more colourful the plate is, the more the kids enjoy their meals. Including seasonal vegetables also helps.
Fruits	All fruits, berries, melons and citrus fruits	They are a power house of antioxidants.	Antioxidants aid in increasing immunity and keep infections at bay.
Fish and poultry	All fatty fish, shell fish, whole eggs, chicken, organ meats	Fatty fish is a good source of Omega 3 fatty acids, shell fish are rich sources of zinc, calcium and other minerals. Whole eggs are high in proteins and vitamin D and zinc.	All these minerals and vitamins are essential for overall growth and avoiding any deficiencies.

Food group	Description	Reason	
Nuts and dried fruits	Almonds, walnuts, pistachios, cashew nuts, figs, dates, raisins	They are a rich source of Omega 3 fatty acids and vitamin E.	They act as a great mid-meal snack and prevent the intake of unnecessary calories from junk foods.
Oils and fats	Butter / cheese/ghee/ mayonnaise	They are among the major nutrients for the development of brain and nervous system. They also help in the absorption of fat soluble vitamins like vitamins A, D, E and K.	Moderation is the key; too much consumption can lead to unnecessary weight gain.

Food group	Description	Reason
Sugar and confectionaries	Table sugar/ maida/ soft drinks	They don't give any particular nutrients, hence the name— empty calories. An occasional indulgence is fine, but these should not replace the above food groups.
Water		An essential nutrient for normal processes in the body. Prevents dehydration and helps avoid constipation.	At least ten to twelve glasses of water every day is a must!

A Teenager's Diet

(Age group: 11–15 years)

This is the age when puberty sets in. During this period of growth spurt, a balanced diet is recommended. The requirement of proteins and nutrients like iron and calcium increases. Iron rich foods like liver, fish, eggs, garden cress seeds, spinach, sprouted pulses, soya bean, dried fruits, etc. are to be included daily. Calcium rich foods like milk and milk products, shell fish, beans and legumes, cereals like ragi and rajgeera, makhana (fox nuts) could provide variety and taste.

Fuel Up: Food Suggestions

Whether you hit the court, the field, the track, the rink, or your backyard to get some physical activity, you'll need some fuel to keep you going!

Here are some great snacks to munch on to keep your body moving and curb hunger pangs:

- Fresh veggies like carrots and celery sticks
- Snack-sized boxes of dry fruits
- Protein bars
- Low-fat yogurt
- Crackers—try graham crackers, animal crackers or saltines
- Local fresh snacks

- Homemade cold sandwiches
- Fruit juice boxes (make sure you choose 100 per cent pure fruit juice, or for an added boost, try orange juice with added calcium)
- Small packages of trail mix

Tip

No matter what type of physical activity you do, you should always be sure to drink plenty of water—before you start, during the activity and after you're done, even if you don't feel thirsty.

Chapter 5

Lifestyle Modification

It's action time! Our previous chapters outlined the factors leading to obesity. The fundamental step towards tackling obesity involves not just losing weight but 'gaining health'—a holistic lifestyle modification.

There are a number of things that shape a child's attitude towards food. If their parents give them money to eat out, they are more likely to buy 'cool' stuff (read junk) instead of salads or fruits. A note to anxious parents who do serve 'healthy' food at home; it must be mentioned here that children have ample access to junk food at their friends' homes or eateries if they are unhappy with the food served at the dining table. Food ordering apps on computers and mobiles also make junk food easily accessible. They are likely to go to their friend's home or a café nearby to buy a sinfully calorie-loaded pastry. If not restrained, children would like to eat ice cream at midnight if only to delay going to bed.

Children would rather eat junk food at the school canteen than carry the 'old-fashioned' chapati-sabzi in their tiffin boxes. The content of tiffin boxes should be 'cool' if one wants to be popular, or so believe many children. In fact, they wouldn't mind carrying crunchy chips or cakes to school in order to win over friends.

There is another aspect to being cool nowadays. With the emergence of social media and the 'influencer' culture, children are being encouraged to eat healthy, feel good and look better. Many popular social media accounts of young men and women talk about holistic food habits but they also reinforce the idea that certain fancy foods like green smoothies, Buddha bowls and other exotic sounding edibles like kale, quinoa, chia, etc., are the way to be if you want to be 'cool'. In 2019, the hashtag '#thestew' made waves globally, which was essentially a chickpea curry made by a popular influencer on Instagram. It was 'trending' as everyone around the globe was making chickpea curries and posting it under the '#thestew'. We never knew that a variation of our humble 'chhole' would be the next hot thing around the world! Similarly, golden latte has taken the world by storm which is otherwise known as 'haldi doodh' in our grandma's kitchen. Suddenly, the boring chhole dal and turmeric milk are hip again.

So, even on social media, there is an imbalance wherein children aspire to get to the cool quotient of eating healthy through fancy super foods like kale, goji berries, asparagus, avocados, dal soups and fruit bowls while they feel that our traditional local Indian food is out of fashion. While the newer generation perhaps wants to make a change, the onslaught of information and popular trends can confuse them.

The child who desires junk food and also the kid who wants to eat healthy but trendy food can be tackled at three levels. The first is at home, as that is the fundamental social unit which plays an important role in shaping a child's beliefs, world views and life choices; the second is the school, as all children take this space of learning seriously. They not only learn the hard skills taught to them through the education system but also various soft skills from their school environment, peers and teachers. The third level to tackle is yourself—the child who has to grow up and become an enthusiastic, productive and responsible adult. How can you do that if you do not live, eat and play the right way? Do you want to be plagued with illnesses that will not allow you to enjoy life to its fullest? So along with your parents and your friends, it's time you make some changes. Read along!

Section 1: Lifestyle Changes at Home

1.　**Let's make meals a family affair and be role-models**

　　While focusing on the child, the rest of the family cannot discard responsibility. Children imitate their parents. Kids learn so much simply by observing others. As a parent, choosing healthier foods and beverages, while limiting the use of electronic devices, may help to reinforce the habits you are trying to encourage in your children. Parents could begin by becoming role models of healthy behaviour—by eating on time, packing a balanced meal and chewing food well.

　　We discussed the 'cool and popular' foods, right? Parents could spend time in making the tiffin box interesting by adding Szechuan sauce to idlis, dosas, rotis and even to vegetables. Store bought Szechuan sauce is laden with salt, sugar and preservatives. You can easily make your own at home. Bhel can be made of boiled sprouts and fruit salads (with ice cream) could replace cartons of readymade juices. Noodles could be liberally peppered with cut vegetables and the nutritious broccoli could serve as a filling in momos.

　　Before the age of 10, children are mouldable and that is the right age to set up these cultures. By making food a family affair, eating healthy can and should be the default programme in every child's brain.

• Dining: Make family meal times a priority

Sometimes, simple acts can have important, long-lasting benefits. According to parenting and health experts, that is exactly the case with family meal times. Eating and talking together helps to foster family unity, improve nutrition, enhance academic success, prevent behavioural problems at home and school, and, most importantly, promote healthy weight among kids. With that impressive list of benefits, it's worth making the time and effort to enjoy more family meal times each week.

It may appear difficult to some to keep up with the varying schedules of different family members, but two family habits go a long way to making all this happen: regular family meals and involving kids in nutrition from the ground up. Begin with incorporating one family meal into the daily schedule. If one family meal per day is not doable, set aside time for a weekend breakfast or lunch. After a month or two of this new pattern, you can add another family meal each week. Before you know it, you will be eating together on most days. Important practices while eating together:

a) Serve medium portions instead of large ones. If a child is hungry after one round of eating, they could take a second serving.
b) Serve regular, balanced meals and snacks with a variety of nutrient rich foods.

c) Explore varied flavours and foods from different cultures and cuisines.

d) Create a routine of pleasant meal times where the family can talk with each other.

e) Remove distractions, such as television, phones and tablets, so that your attention is on each other.

f) Allow children to use their intuition to decide how much and what to eat from the foods you set out for each meal.

2. Let kids help in the kitchen

Young children have a willingness to learn and a genuine desire to help. Cooking together and including children in the food preparation process is a great way to introduce them to holistic choices and practices. The process of healthy food selection will create an awareness of the importance of nutrients, their specific functions and food safety methods, among other things. Assign simple tasks like setting the table or tearing lettuce leaves for a salad, and use the time together to make conversation about the importance of eating home-made food. The idea is to guide children to make healthy choices independently.

Secondly, shopping for food together is a fun activity. Divide food into groups: grains, fruits, vegetables, dairy and protein foods. Children can choose new foods they want to try, including picking out a new fresh/frozen/canned or dried fruit during each trip. As children get older, they can help plan the menu at home and then pick out the foods to match the menu items while shopping. The advantage of cooking meals and involving children is that the parent and child are both mindful of nutrition and portions. While we discussed becoming aware of how each food item, fruit, vegetable and grain affects the body, you can talk to your child on similar lines when you shop for food and cook together. It is not feasible to offload a ton of information on the child like a school syllabus. But the child has to be initiated into practices with small doses of information over a period of time.

For example, if you go to a super-market, you could shop for ingredients to bake cake or cookies. While the conventional recipe calls for refined wheat or maida you could tell your child to buy whole-wheat and oat-flour as a substitute as it is healthier. You could slowly swap sugar for jaggery and so on. When you make these changes, ensure that you talk to the child about such small but significant changes. And let's be honest, substituting maida with a whole-grain and sugar with jaggery is a matter of discipline; because cakes with refined flour and white sugar are more palatable than their healthier counterparts. So in a way, the child will pick up that they are being restricted from certain 'goodies'. To compensate, let them have a free hand in choosing fruits that can go into your baked goods. That way, you are disciplining them and at the same time offering them freedom to make healthier choices.

It is only when one is cooking, do they realize the quantity of sugar, fat and salt that goes into any recipe versus when a cook has made it or when it has been ordered from a restaurant. It is only when we bake a cake that we realize the quantity of sugar and butter that we consume with every serving. Else, that single, seemingly innocent and tiny piece from a whole cake seems pretty harmless, doesn't it? It is only when you take control of the kitchen that you realize the implications of that tiny piece of cake or that extra spoon of sugar. Similarly, once the child starts participating in cooking activities, they will be better informed to make smarter food choices in the long run.

There are also other ways you can use to make your children practice healthier lifestyles on a day-to-day basis. You could grow a garden! While it may seem unconventional and drastic, it could be an activity your children and you respond to. The process of planting, watching over and harvesting a garden can provide children with many valuable lessons. It becomes a physical activity, teaches them to care for and understand the value of living things and also allows them a sense of control in growing their own food.

3. Eating in versus eating out

Here are three typical scenarios that I encounter consistently in my practice:

Scene 1: In the life of a busy urban working couple, say in Mumbai, the routine of the day is like clockwork: early mornings, long commutes, high work pressures and so on. Typically, a house help is appointed to take care of home chores like cleaning and cooking so that some of their workload can be outsourced. When the child leaves for school in the morning, there are times when they are handed money to eat from school canteens as the early morning cooking session has been skipped. Or else, often an unsupervised cook has prepared lunch boxes for the entire family. I say this because on an everyday basis, we can't control the oil content or the sauces the cook would add based on their judgement to create 'tasty' food. Often, breakfasts are quick or skipped. When the child returns home from school to an empty fridge, parents are likely to order in some tasty snack from a food app (where previously someone would have home cooked it for the child). When parents pick up the kid from an activity class, they might say, 'I don't have time to cook dinner, let's eat out.' This leads to the child and family consuming high-calorie, high-fat food multiple times a week.

Scene 2: In the newly developing towns of our country, thanks to the media flux, house parties have been converted into restaurant treats. Parties and family get-togethers that were once home catered, now take place in halls or on restaurant tables. I see this also as a trend in lower economic groups in the city. One is aware of the detrimental repercussions of reused oil, tastemakers and ingredients like monosodium glutamate (MSG). Also notice the high number of 'jhunka bhakar kendras' and roadside Chinese food stalls that facilitate quick lunches and dinners for these suburban families.

Scene 3: Many of my affluent patients showcase a distaste for our traditional or, if I may say so, 'basic' Indian meals. They feel that 'sabzi roti' is a poor man's food! Their taste is exotic and global—cheesy pizzas and pastas have replaced the food of their ancestors. In fact, many children I know hate Indian food in their lunch boxes. They want 'cool' food, which also leads them to eat out often.

In all three scenarios, you may argue, eating out is inevitable owing to schedules or social circumstances. Don't we all recall how we loved home-cooked meals? There were particular recipes our mothers made that were a huge hit amongst our friends. Weren't our birthday parties and get-togethers filled with home-made meals? I remember how my friends' mothers would ask my mom for certain recipes that their child liked. Naysayers might say to me that I am living in a fantasy world if I think parents are going to start cooking dinner again. But I strongly assert that we have to revert to our basics because home-cooked food is the best way to control fat and sugar.

I understand that for children especially, refusing to eat out seems impossible. But we can develop certain habits that can help them in the long run. For example, while eating out, you can talk about how portion sizes have grown bigger than in the past. Make it a rule to share entrées or have the child eat an appetizer as their main course. Turn down the bread basket, order salads, avoid rich sauces and share or skip dessert. If you follow my previous advice of cooking meals with your child, they will develop a relationship with food where they do not feel that a chef's cooking is superior to home-cooked meals. As a practice, you and your child could recreate restaurant meals of their choice. It is a slow and cultural process to make them perceive food not merely as a treat but as the only vital source of nutrition.

4. Body positivity

'Do you want to walk like that person?'
'Do you want to become as ugly as them?'
'You will never get selected for sports.'

These are commonly used statements to scare children into exercising or eating healthy. As parents and adults, when we are trying to explain the consequences of obesity to children, we tend to show them obese individuals on television, or even worse, in public areas or give an example of an overweight relative, uncle, cousin, grandparent or friend and scare them into imagining their life if they looked like them! But what is the message that you are sending? You are not telling them to be fit for health reasons but to avoid being in situations where they get mocked or become social outcasts.

Being obese is not an indicator of anyone's character or traits. It is just a physical condition or an ailment like a cough, cold or fever. This is why it is imperative that we do not belittle or make fun of or judge people who are overweight, when teaching our children to be health conscious. Parents should be careful about the language and context they use to describe overweight persons. Never talk about an overweight person in a negative manner.

It is also important that we check the way we speak to people who appear overweight to us. It is common to advise a seemingly 'fat' person on their weight publicly even when we have no information about their medical history. These occurrences are common and look like they are genuine concerns from well-wishers. Everyone's weight is their personal matter and they are well aware of its consequences. Suggesting that an overweight person needs to 'work harder' or 'not be lazy' or 'have more willpower' or 'eat less' is a breach of their privacy and space. They could be suffering from certain medical conditions, certain medications, genetics, etc.

Our society feels it is okay to talk or comment on someone's weight, advise them and even shame them for it. Children will pick up the prejudices you leave around. It could lead to the child developing an inferiority complex if they feel that they are overweight or it could lead to them believing that obesity is a vice. They will believe that 'fat' is a bad word and not the symptom of an illness.

There is also the media that has and continues to portray overweight people in a negative light; that they are silly, unintelligent and lazy, or at times, even vicious bullies. Parents have to be sensitive of the media the child is getting exposed to, as a lot of cartoons and television shows and series portray overweight people as individuals to be made fun of. How often do you remember a plus-size model or an actor being portrayed as a regular person? This influences the perception and attitudes of obese children and of other children towards them. Seeing an obese person should serve as a reminder that obesity is a disease and prevention could just be the best cure.

5. Taming screen time

Television can take a toll on your child's nutrition. Watching television while eating increases eating portions and commercials have an added negative implication. Advertisements are designed in a such way that they draw people to their products. This is especially true in the case of impressionable children when it comes to food.

Each day, while watching television, children between the ages of 10 and 13 are exposed to advertisements that promote a food or beverage. A majority of these advertisements do not meet the nutrition recommendations established by several government agencies. Many foods shown in commercials do not contribute to their growing brains and bodies. Many are high in solid fats, added sugars, sodium and/or calories and often lack vitamins, minerals and dietary fibre.

So how can you tame these temptations on television and promote healthier eating? **Avoid watching** television **while eating!** As a family, agree not to watch television (or use other electronic devices) during meals or while snacking. Designate a few areas, such as the dining table or beds, as no-screen zones. Alternately, pick up a time (say 5–7 p.m.) when all screens are banned. Eating together regularly sans distractions also promotes mindful eating and family bonding.

Watch children's programmes without advertisements. Consider a streaming service subscription for children that does away with commercials. The American Academy of Pediatrics recommends no more than one hour per day of screen time for children between 2 and 5 years of age and the use of a family media plan for school-age children.

6. Bedtime

Bedtime is sacrosanct. Adequate sleep is almost as important as nutrition to stay healthy. Stick to a fixed bed time and keep electronics away from the bed. Fatigue leads to overeating and can prime the body for weight gain. Overweight children may need treatment for sleep apnoea as well. When you do not sleep enough, your inflammatory markers increase and raise blood pressure, insulin and cortisol levels. Hence, children should be told that they should get on to their beds by, say, 10 p.m., without their phone or tabs.

7. Let's play

One of the key aspects that I want to focus on as a lifestyle is the culture of outdoor play. Engaging in regular physical activity helps fight obesity. Ideally, children should engage in a minimum of sixty minutes of moderate to vigorous intensity physical activity each day. It should involve outdoor and indoor activities. Parents play an important role in encouraging kids in being physically active.

Section 2: At School

Schools could play a vital role by promoting healthy food ideas to children even while conveying the cons of being obese. The foundation for lifelong good health is laid in childhood. Outside of home life, nothing provides more of an immersive experience for children than the time they spend in school. This means that schools have a rich opportunity to improve the health of the youth and tackle obesity at the ideal point in time before problems take hold.

One of the main avenues that schools can use to positively affect health is also directly in line with every school's mission: educating students. Nutrition and physical activity lessons can be inculcated into the curriculum in core classroom subjects, physical education and after-school programmes to teach skills that help students choose and maintain healthy lifestyles. In addition to teaching evidence-based nutrition and activity lessons, the school's physical education should focus on getting students engaged in high quality and regular activity.

Schools can also promote health outside of the classroom by surrounding students with opportunities to eat healthy and stay active. To improve nutrition, schools can include healthier food offerings in the cafeteria and eliminate marketing of unhealthy foods. To improve activity, schools can develop safe walking and biking routes to school, and can promote active recess time.

Wellness programmes for faculty and staff can also be integral to improving the school environment. They will not only boost faculty and staff health but also build enthusiasm for student-focused programmes across the institute.

Additionally, schools can serve as important data sources on student health. Anonymous, school-level information on markers like students' BMI can help educators and policymakers assess the success of ongoing programmes and decide the direction of future programmes.

With good evidence that school-based prevention programmes can successfully and without too many added resources help students eat better, be more active and achieve healthier weights, schools are poised to become an integral part of the fight against the obesity epidemic. As with education in general, the sooner we act, the better.

Serving healthy choices in the lunch room, limiting the availability and marketing of unhealthful foods and sugary drinks, and making water available to students throughout the day are some of the ways that schools can help prevent obesity.

Making these types of changes in the school food environment will be no easy task. However, countries across the world are working on this. For example, in the US, the Michelle Obama initiative—Choose My Plate—drove institutions like schools and colleges to introspect on food choices. Also, as the initiative's website had effectively consolidated all the information needed to make these choices, the institutions used it as a tool to further awareness. Also, at a macro level, the USDA recently finalized comprehensive new school meal guidelines that will increase vegetables, fruit and whole grains, and curb sodium, saturated fat and trans fat. But due to political pressures, the agency was not able to fully implement the meal guidelines recommended by an expert panel at the Institute of Medicine. The Eat Well Guide issued by the UK government is another such tool to establish knowledge about food and correct eating methods at various levels, be it homes or schools.

I understand that schools may face many other challenges in creating a food environment where the healthy choice is the default choice. Some of these obstacles may be: budgeting for the higher costs of purchasing and preparing more healthful foods; coaxing children to accept the healthy options; and addressing the multitude of ways that unhealthy foods and drinks are sold or served outside of school meals, from classroom birthday parties to school-wide bake sales and sporting events. However, I urge the right institutions to join this fight against obesity so that our children don't become Generation XL.

Japan, the country with one of the lowest obesity rates, has managed to successfully implement the School Lunch Act in its legal framework. Kyushoku or school lunches serve delicious lunch and food lessons to students. Kyushoku translates to 'meals provided by institutions like schools and companies'. In Japanese schools, Kyushoku is a part of the curriculum where students take turns to help set up lunches, serve food to fellow students and eat together once everyone is served. Children are allowed to talk, foster warmth, togetherness and relax during the break time but they are also expected to follow discipline and table manners. The children clean up after themselves, stacking their plates and wheeling them back to the kitchen where the staff washes them.

Students are also taught important lessons on no wastage, picky eating is discouraged and the school nutritionist takes feedback that is implemented in upcoming meals. Schools have qualified nutritionists who oversee meals and ensure that children get well-balanced and wholesome meals. The food is prepared from scratch with raw ingredients that are grown locally. The children are made aware of farming practices: cultivating, harvesting, processing and so on. It is emphasized that food is harvested and acquired from living beings, and hence, it should be treated with respect and gratitude. The payoff is that the children are healthier, happier and imbibe holistic food habits.

You may argue that this system can be followed in 'rich' and 'elite' schools because practices such as hiring a dietician, growing and procuring local ingredients and so on require significant capital. But in Japan, Kyushoku is successfully implemented across the country because the government supports and endorses it. Since it was introduced in 1954, the School Lunch Act has witnessed many amendments, which introduced various food groups into school lunches, set up subsidies, established dietary leadership, etc. In 2005, the Shokuiku Basic Act was enacted to legislate food education. In 2008, the School Lunch Act was revised to amend the goals of school lunches as per the Shokuiku Basic Act. Finally, in 2009, the revised School Lunch Act was implemented, the benefits and success of which are evident. The bottom line is that health is not a prerogative of the rich but a fundamental right that can be made available to all if the government and higher authorities act upon it.

Another important aspect is physical activity. As mentioned earlier, children require at least sixty minutes of moderate-to-vigorous-intensity physical activity each day. Though PE is an important part of all school curriculums, we know that many children do not participate. The reasons? Well, some children who are not 'sporty' decide to recede to the fringes and chat with each other. When the session involves coaching, there is a lot of time spent waiting, without much physical activity, for one's turn. Sometimes, children who are fat shamed or may be introverts and shy, don't want to participate. And sometimes, in urban schools, especially in cities like

Mumbai, there is not enough space. Many such reasons prevent students from benefiting from physical activity classes in school. However, let us take a step to tackle this at the institutional level.

A quick list of some essentials that the school can definitely implement to begin with include:

- Encouraging students to participate in breakfast, lunch and after-school snack programmes so that their involvement and knowledge increases.

- A short film or talk on the dire consequences of being obese—right from not being able to be as active as one would like to be to carrying a higher risk for diseases such as blood pressure, diabetes and cancer—should be periodically shown to children when they are studying in lower classes. The school must ensure that the activity is sensitive and empathetic towards those suffering from obesity and the individual is not singled out or bullied.

- Investing in cafeteria facilities to store, prepare and display healthy foods, such as salad bars. Set minimum and maximum calorie levels for school breakfast and lunch for each age group. Train food service staff in healthy food preparation techniques and food safety.

- Giving students adequate time to eat.

- Incorporating nutrition education and physical education into school meal programmes.

- Ensuring that competitive foods meet healthy nutrition standards that are consistent with those of the school meal programme. Eliminate artificially sweetened beverages from the school environment or limit access to them.

- Ensuring that food served at classroom parties and school functions meets nutritional food standards set by the school.

- Not using food as a reward or punishment.

- Making drinking water freely available to students in dining areas and throughout the day.

- Creating pleasant, clean and safe cafeterias.

- Prohibiting commercial food marketing outside of dining areas.

- Prohibiting marketing of foods that do not meet competitive food guidelines or other nutrition standards; or prohibiting all food advertising in schools.

- Creating and supporting school gardens.

- Encouraging staff to model healthy eating.

- Encouraging students to stay active throughout the school day.

- Providing all students with opportunities for daily physical activity.

- Developing active transit plans (bike, walk to school), in collaboration with local governments and community groups. Also, offer children physical activity opportunities before and after school, including competitive sports and non-competitive activities. Collaborate with communities to maximize use of school and community spaces for physical activity during and outside school hours.

- Offering staff opportunities for physical activity.

Chapter 6

Exercise

A physically active child is a healthy child. Keeping your children active should be a priority for their health and well-being.

Every parent wants their children to grow up strong and healthy. One of the factors that makes children healthy is their level of exercise and fitness and how consistent they are.

Regular physical activity helps your child develop in a range of ways. Not only does it help their physical health, but it also helps improve their brain function and emotional wellbeing.

The earlier the child starts getting in shape, the risk of obesity reduces even further.

Research indicates that inactive children are likely to become inactive adults, putting young people at risk of developing life-threatening conditions.

Exercise is a key part of life in the young. Unlike adults, children do not have a designated time for exercise. Instead exercise is part of their life. A child plays at school, at home and in the community.

Exercises are diverse, ranging from individual and team sporting activities, extracurricular activities such as dancing and many more. When a child is physically fit, he or she feels and looks better.

There are various benefits of moderate exercise in a child.

It keeps the calories in check. Sedentary is the new smoking is my favourite joke in seminars. Exercises helps maintain a leaner shape, improves fitness and reduces the risk of obesity in adulthood.

Like other muscles in our body, the heart is one of the most relentlessly worked muscles. Its performance improves when it is regularly challenged by exercise by becoming stronger and more efficient. Thus, warding off heart diseases which are rampantly becoming common in young individuals. Through this, it helps keep our arteries and veins clear of harmful cholesterol, reducing the risk of cardiovascular diseases. More blood circulation increases the flexibility of the blood vessels wall and therefore reduces high blood pressure.

We all have learnt what oxygen saturation (SpO2) means and the importance of it in this pandemic, among many things. SpO2 directly links to the lungs' capacity and their efficiency in moving air in and out of the body.

Regular exercise helps maintain that capacity and therefore provides a large amount of oxygen in the body that helps in multiple ways.

It reduces blood sugar levels and the risks of Type 2 diabetes. Insulin, which regulates sugars in an individual, is directly affected by the level of exercise and diet a child follows.

Just as muscles grow stronger, bones too respond to regular exercises by getting stronger. Increased bone density helps prevent diseases related to your knees and back, which is commonly seen in obese adults.

It helps prevent cancer. Incidences of cancer of colon, breast and prostrate are far lower.

In pubescent girls, aside from providing general physical benefits, regular activity can also help ease symptoms of premenstrual syndrome. This is because moderate exercise helps the body produce hormones called endorphins. These are natural painkillers that can ease cramps and back pain as well as improve mood.

Along with these aforementioned benefits on the organs, the most undermined organ is the brain in my opinion, specially in our community and the lifestyle it demands.

Physical activity plays an important role in developing the brain and supporting essential mental functions.

Exercise leads to improved motor skills (such as hand-eye co-ordination), better thinking and problem solving, stronger attention skills and improved learning. Studies say physical activity allows children to have a better outlook on life by building confidence, managing anxiety and depression and increasing self-esteem and cognitive skills.

The effect of exercise on the brain is of three kinds.

The immediate effect on the brain is evident by the secretion of dopamine, serotonin and noradrenaline. These are your happy hormones, which help you elevate your mood. Studies correlate high levels of endorphins in happy children. Hence physical activities may serve as a complementary treatment to treat depression/anxiety in children, something which doctors, psychologists, PE teachers and importantly parents agree on. Children with aggravated anxiety focus on whatever makes them anxious, which in turn makes them more anxious and keeps the cycle going. With exercise, the child can break this cycle, develop a new skill and achieve a sense of accomplishment.

Psychologists are not only using physical activity to prevent mental and physical illness but also treat other conditions, including grief, heartache, bad moods, and ease relationships and family counselling. If a child or a teen is feeling lonely, a team activity can give them a sense of belonging and companionship. A sport provides relief from social pressure. Sharing experiences with peers, developing relationships and working towards a common goal always enable a child to focus. It also encourages them to speak in public, which many would otherwise find difficult.

Children with conditions such as bipolar disorder or schizophrenia have shown positive responses to exercise.

Those suffering from mental health issues might find it challenging to follow a programme of physical exercise. However, the child will benefit if the right guidance is provided. The mental energy used in creating disruptions is instead dissipated in physical activity.

Secondly, the anatomy and brain physiology change after following an exercise programme.

Studies indicate that the volume of the hippocampus (the most fascinating part of the brain, in my opinion) shows an increase in patients after they follow a year-long exercise programme consistently. This proves that with increased blood circulation due to exercise, the brain develops, just as muscles do, thus benefitting long-term memory. Those who exercise have an increased attention span by two hours compared to sedentary individuals.

Third, exercise has a protective effect. The pre-frontal cortex also enlarges, along with the hippocampus, due to exercise. Both the hippocampus and pre-frontal cortex are helpful in detecting neurodegenerative diseases and ageing. Exercise delays the onset of Parkinson's disease and amnesia in those individuals with strong familial traits for these conditions.

'Agreed Doc, but how can I get my child to work out more?' or worse 'I think my child is physically active enough in school.'

These are the few hurdles that are thrown at me when I ask them about the quantity and quality of their child's physical activity.

Here's my advice. Firstly, it is very imperative to introspect. We, as adults, play a very important role indirectly, whether we like it or not. Being that 'healthy role model' will not just help them stay physically active but mentally fit too. I have always encouraged parents to take part in their children's physical activities, to whatever extent it is permitted. One of the best ways to do this is by initiating a habit of activity yourself and include your children in it. An everyday example is taking the stairs or walking instead of opting for public transport or private cars for running errands. It is more challenging to motivate your child to participate in regular exercise if you don't lead by example. This is especially true when you spend your time on your computer or mobile. The child follows suit subconsciously.

Create a positive environment. Due to social pressure, trends and many other social constructs, it is easy for us to judge. Judging leads to negative reinforcement. We tend to criticize the child for not working out or being more physically active. This does not leave the child feeling good, thus forcing them to seek comfort in food and other unwanted avenues.

The 'one size fits all' surely does not apply here or in every aspect of tackling this issue. An assessment of your child is imperative.

Harsh, the neighbour's kid, will have an aptitude for a different sport or approach to your Nikhil.

Your attitude towards the activity will be projected on to your child's wellbeing and their approach to it. Physical literacy is an unheard of concept, let alone emphasised.

It is important to encourage the child to find an activity that they enjoy. Keeping it fun should be the mantra here. So it does not become a chore and gains the child's interest, thus ensuring that the child sticks to it. The type varies from one individual to another. It can either be team-led or going to a nearby sporting club for lessons in swimming or tennis. Dance is a great form of exercise and commonly shunned, due to gender bias. After assessment of your child's likes and dislikes, understand the importance of variety in the child's exercise. If you examine children on the playground, one should look out for these three components: endurance, strength and flexibility.

A child builds endurance when they regularly get aerobic activity, using the large muscles, making the heart beat faster and increasing the respiratory rate. They can be in the form of cricket, basketball, football, hockey, tennis, track and field (running or jumping) and swimming.

Strength can be assessed by the distance your child travels on the monkey bar.

Improving strength does not necessarily mean lifting weights. A few simple push ups, sit ups and pull ups can easily improve strength. Covid has made us realize the importance of home gyms. Simple home gym set-ups are feasible with basic equipment and any financial budgets.

The final component that is assessed is flexibility. If the child bends down to tie their shoelaces and how they do it is a good everyday tool. Other assessments include reaching out for toys or performing cartwheels or splits.

Now the questions arises, how much exercise is enough? The amount depends on the child's age.

For children under 5 years, who are not yet walking, physical activity is any movement.

For example, children this age enjoy floor-based play in different positions; this could include 'tummy time', rolling on the ground or reaching for toys. Water-based activities are excellent. One should ensure there is good balance of activity and rest. Minimize long periods of time in the same position, such as time strapped into car seats or carriers, and time spent in front of a TV or other screens.

Children under 5 years, who are walking by themselves, should be active for at least a total of 180 minutes (3 hours/day). This does not have to be all at once, so their physical activity can be spread throughout the day.

Physical activity can be unstructured active play or structured exercise of varying intensities. Movement skills gained at this young age set the scene for movement skills, such as balance and coordination, when older.

Children this age should not be inactive for long periods of time, except for when they are asleep. So minimize time spent watching TV, on computer games or time spent in a push chair.

Children and young people of 5–18 years should take part in moderate to vigorous physical activities for at least 60 minutes (one hour) every day, and this can be up to several hours. Moderate intensity activity means working hard enough to raise your heartbeat, so you breathe harder and begin to sweat, but are still able to talk. Vigorous intensity activity means that your heart rate and breathing are harder and faster and talking is more difficult.

Your child should be doing higher intensity and resistance activities three days a week, as these will help to strengthen muscles and bones.

Children and young people of all ages should avoid spending long periods sitting down without moving.

Schools and school selection also play an integral part in the child's daily physical activities.

Along with the academic pedigree of the school, their approach to physical education and other school-related topics should be equally considered.

They can be broadly categorized into:

- Physical education
- Active transportation
- Activity breaks
- The school's physical environment
- After-school intervention

PE provides students the opportunity to obtain the knowledge and skills needed to establish and maintain a physically active lifestyle through childhood and adolescence and into adulthood. PE can enhance students' knowledge and skills about why and how they should be physically active, therefore establishing physical literacy.

A newer approach is characterized by a focus on increasing overall physical activity, particularly moderate to vigorous intensity physical activity, during PE class.

Enhanced PE is characterized by the following components:

- Increasing the amount of time students spend in moderate-to-vigorous intensity physical activity during PE lessons.
- Adding more physical education classes to the school curriculum.
- Lengthening the time of existing physical education classes.
- Meeting the physical activity needs of all students, including those with disabilities.
- Including activities that are enjoyable for students while emphasising knowledge and skills that can be used for a lifetime.
- Educating and encouraging parents to participate with their children in active transportation to school.

Activity Breaks

The school setting can offer opportunities for students to participate in and enjoy physical activity outside of

PE class, including recess and physical activity within the classroom. Such opportunities are referred to as activity breaks. Most often, the overarching strategy behind activity breaks has been to establish an environment that promotes regular physical activity throughout the school day. This can occur through regularly scheduled recess and lunch time physical activity or by implementing 5- to 10-minute breaks during classroom time that may or may not include subject matter curriculum.

Chapter 7

Therapy

Indian society has a very straightforward approach to food. We love food. As mentioned before, a belly equates to wealth and health in the community, with no age bar. However, with rapid globalization and modernization, this may not be true anymore. With the Gen Z culture on the horizon, millennials are overly self-conscious and often obsess over the idealized body parading about on their social media platforms. As a parent, you've always made sure that your child is well fed, insisted on that third, sometimes even fourth, helping. But suddenly they are trying to explain what calorie deficit or weight cutting is, which sounds as absurd as the next fad diet. Then the self-conscious pre-teen compounds with the dreaded question of 'Am I fat?', leaving you even more gobsmacked. This question either provokes silence or complete denial from a parent. Even a carefully phrased response may lead to an unwarranted eating disorder.

That's a tricky situation, no?

Here are my two cents. The goal should be to find a balance between reality and idealism.

Firstly, a parent should not overreact when put on the spot.

Teasing and bullying of overweight or chubby children is endemic in our school and society. It is apparent in our movies; it is apparent in our daily engagements.

If the child has mentioned it, the issue is not going away and a conversation where the child does the talking will give you a better perspective on how to deal with the situation.

Most overweight children do not lose weight without an adult's aid. For instance, we do not expect them to learn to read without being taught.

Do not label them lazy or make them feel guilty about their eating habits. Scaring or bribing the child to lose weight is not the best option either. And lastly, avoid the easiest way out—deflecting or joking about weight gain or increased sizes.

It is not what you say, it is the way you say it. It is about encouraging self-discovery, uniqueness and individuality in our children.

Keeping it casual is the theme that I recommend.

Do everything as a family. Move as a unit. Change as a unit. It is helpful to focus the conversation on the entire family as opposed to a specific child. Discussion should be open on the dinner table, involving every member of the family. Introduce concepts such as 'eating healthy is important to our family so we all can live long lives'. Parents should focus their conversations on their child's health behaviours rather than weight, shape or size. Keeping the focus on health helps the child have a better idea of what 'to do' versus 'not to do'. As aforementioned, along with physical literacy, dietary literacy is equally important.

Try to guide and not control your child's eating habits. Many eating disorders involve a feeling of not being in control. If we create a casual environment, our sons and daughters develop normally, without interference.

To treat any food disorder, the first thing that is taught is that food is neutral. There is no healthy food or unhealthy food. Otherwise, these connotations lead to morality around food, terming the child 'bad' if they happen to indulge. This leads to a cycle of longing for forbidden food and then feeling shame when we do eat it, making secrecy the biggest problem around food. Controlling works to a limited degree, when the child mostly eats at home. But in the community, and, more importantly, in school, they tend to act out and binge on junk.

Children up to the age of 7 have little direct control over what they eat and how they spend their time. Your child's weight can be managed by monitoring their access to sugary and fatty foods.

Primary school-age children (7–11) have the opportunity to make more choices about what they eat and what they do. Managing weight during these years usually involves some degree of co-operation between parent and child. Because of this, it can be helpful for parents to talk to their children about why they are being asked to eat fewer unhealthy foods.

Adolescents (age 12 onwards) have quite sophisticated views about nutrition and health, and strong feelings about whether or not they like the look of their bodies at a heavier weight. They have more (but not total) responsibility for the food that they eat and how they spend their time. They can understand the idea of managing weight, and with support, can come up with creative ideas about this.

The intervention of a nutritionist when required is always encouraged. Like it is said, 'It takes a village to raise a child.'

It is heart-wrenching to tell ten-year-olds that they cannot eat a cheese 'pav bhaji' owing to obesity and must follow a diet. But due diligence to diet is imperative and parents, doctors and dieticians must ideally find ways around such situations to maintain gradual and long-lasting progress.

There will definitely come a point in the exercise when the child is so emotionally drained by the monotony of a diet and hectic physical activities that the treatment will stop having a positive impact. Over the years, I have realized that people lose up to 10 per cent of their initial weight with the most stringent diets. This is seen in adults, who are committed to losing weight, and not children, who don't fully comprehend the concept.

It is at this saturation point that doctors may feel the need to push the patient to the next step and introduce cognitive behavioural therapy (CBT) that could act as a catalyst for weight loss. For the uninitiated, CBT entails 'talking' in such a manner that it changes the way a patient thinks and behaves. While it is commonly used in mental health to treat depression and anxiety disorders, it is known to help people with physical health problems as well. Obesity is one area where CBT has shown results in the last few decades.

A study from the Netherlands has shown that CBT helps obese children reduce their BMI score, which is the measuring scale for obesity. This study looked at the effects of a family-based CBT on eighty children who were aged between 8 and 17 years. The children were divided into two groups with one group receiving CBT and the other getting the standard diet-and-exercise regimen. Over two years, the children attended group sessions for periods of three months at a stretch. The group that received CBT had significantly reduced its BMI. I am mentioning the details so that parents and teenagers realize that every intervention takes hard work, commitment and, above all, time. There are, unfortunately, no quick-fixes or magic bullets to stop obesity's march.

CBT for obesity works on the principle that an obese person has 'maladapted eating and exercise patterns' and these behaviours can be modified to achieve weight loss. Before diets and medicines became popular two decades ago, CBT was the mainstay for an individual's weight reduction initiatives.

The psychologist or behaviour therapist not only talks to change the child's feelings vis-à-vis food, but also gives some practical tips that could increase the effectiveness of the weight loss diet and exercises. Many therapists, for instance, advise teenagers to maintain a 'food diary' where they can write down details about their meals, the calories they tucked in and so on. In case of younger children, parents could help them with this task.

Usually, children are asked to choose a goal—say they want to lose five kilos in six months or ten kilos at the end of the year. Not only does the setting up of a goal post make the monitoring process interesting, it also makes children feel that they are achieving something worthwhile.

Stimulus control is another important pillar of CBT in obesity management. Parents would be advised to alter the environment at home so that no one, especially the child, eats in excess. Smaller serving dishes than the usual could be put on the dining table and the amount of food served on each plate could be less than before. Due to CBT, the child will hesitate before seeking a second or third helping, thereby controlling the urge (or the stimulus) to overeat.

Children should be taught to chew their food slowly and should be rewarded for eating well or regularly updating their food diary. CBT also teaches the child the ills of overeating and its link to obesity.

A study published in the *European Journal of Clinical Nutrition* in 2007 showed that CBT worked even after five years among some children. While a third of the children dropped out of the aforesaid study, those who stuck around managed to reduce their BMI, decrease their waist circumference and could manage their movements better.

In India too, my fellow bariatric surgeons and endocrinologists have acknowledged that positive, persistent results can be obtained in obese children by combining a lifestyle-centred approach where the parents are involved along with nutritional and cognitive behavioural strategies. I would say most obese children and teenagers can be managed with this combination of diet, exercise and cognitive therapy.

For a small section of patients, the doctors may need to go the next step that involves introducing an oral medicine to optimize losing weight.

Part 3

Chapter 8

The Last Resort: Bariatric Surgery

History of Bariatric Surgery

The relative safety of bariatric procedures today stands in stark contrast to the measures adopted by those living in the mid-twentieth century. Obesity has historically been perceived as a sign of affluence and wealth, but the onset of mercantile economies has made food a widely available commodity. More food means more people eating food, and more people eating too much food is an inevitable consequence of surplus availability for cheap prices.

This led to the first informal technique that attempted to control excessive weight in people. This method was jaw wiring, wherein the jaw was wired shut to reduce food intake. However, this method failed due to several difficulties. Besides the obvious flaw in logic, those who had gotten their jaws wired struggled to maintain their dental health and suffered various issues with oral hygiene. Furthermore, while it prevented food intake, it did not prevent the ingestion of high calorific liquids. This ensured the failure of jaw wiring as a procedure, but it did bring to light an important issue: the need for corrective procedures to reduce the risk of obesity.

The next major procedure to be attempted was the jejunoileal bypass. This is the first technique that did not rely on restriction, but on malabsorption, which is the reduction in amount of nutrients absorbed by the small intestines. While this procedure did cause significant weight loss, it also led to several horrifying complications in almost all the patients who pursued it. These included diarrhoea, skin problems, severe arthritis, night blindness, osteoporosis, malnutrition, kidney stones, liver failure and flu-like symptoms. Some variations of this procedure, such as the jejunocolic bypass and others, were also successful in catalysing weight loss, but they too caused major complications that led to these techniques dying out.

After these failures, medical practitioners struck gold when the gastric bypass was popularized in the 1960s. Over the decades, this procedure would become one of, if not the most popular bariatric surgeries in the world. During this period, it has seen changes in the way the procedure is carried out and a massive reduction in resulting complications, making it one of the safest procedures available today. Following the invention of the gastric bypass, the biliopancreatic diversion was first popularized without a duodenal switch, and later with it. The innovation regarding surgical techniques continues till date, with surgeons constantly looking to improve old procedures and construct new ones. The specifics of these procedures are covered in the following sections.

For severe cases, medicines are effective only as a complementary measure to lifestyle modification. In contrast, bariatric surgery has recently gained prominence as an excellent procedure for the obese. Anyone who requires this procedure has assuredly contracted some of the chronic illnesses that accompany obesity. Surgery not only helps patients bring their weight down to a healthier level, but also heals these chronic illnesses, such as hypertension, diabetes, infertility and others. This, in turn, also soothes the anxiety and depression caused by being overweight. The result is a tremendously positive impact on the lives of those who have seen the worst of this disease. It has been found that bariatric surgery reduces up to one-third of the patients' pre-operative weight, and this loss remains stable for years after, unlike what has been observed with alternative therapies.

That this procedure can be offered to infants and toddlers is a testimony to the marvel that is modern medical science. I once operated on an infant named Zoya from Mumbai, who was less than twelve-months-old on the day of the procedure. While extreme precaution must be exercised before operating on babies, some cases deem it absolutely unavoidable. These mainly include instances where obesity is a result of genetic mutation. Zoya weighed nineteen kilos despite being less than a year old. Normally, a three to four year old weighs that much. Besides genetics, another factor that makes surgery a viable option for children is the observation that measures like dietary restrictions, lifestyle modification and increased physical activity are better suited to adults. Research shows that the more someone weighs, the less likely it is that lifestyle modification will benefit them. A third aspect is the fact that a child's struggles with weight may also be dependent on the marital status and health of the parents. For example, it has been found that children whose parents are slim and married, lose weight easier than those with obese, divorced or separated parents.

All of these reasons, and the progress of medicine, have enabled children to be the lucky beneficiaries of bariatric surgery. Yet, the question of operating on children is fraught with ethical dilemmas for two main reasons. Firstly, benefits aside, bariatric surgery is *not* a long-term solution. Those that are obese due to abnormal genes will likely need to undergo the procedure at least once more in their lifetime. Zoya required a second surgery eight years after her first one. This is because these genes ensure that obese children never feel full, regardless of the amount of food they eat, encouraging overeating, and consequently, gaining weight. Furthermore, only a small percentage—between 2 and 6 per cent—of obese patients develop the disease during early childhood. Surgically operating on these children will not help in the long run. In addition to this, the process of gaining a doctor's approval for surgery can be long drawn out and tedious. On consulting a surgeon in India, an obese child is subjected to a barrage of tests to determine any genetic influence on their weight.

These samples are sent abroad for testing, and a diagnosis is obtained only after several months have passed. Meanwhile, the child is put on a liquid diet and provided medicines, depending on the severity of the case and the age of the patient. Developmental milestones, such as walking, are also considered. Is obesity hampering their ability to walk and how serious is the obstruction? Answers to these questions, and the child's response to medicines and the diet, are gauged in determining the need for surgery. Depending on these factors, a child may or may not even qualify for the procedure. In a study on this, half of the 750 paediatricians interviewed in the US revealed that they would never refer even adolescents for surgery, let alone children. Even if the child meets the requirements and undergoes the surgery, they will need to follow up with a team of doctors for at least two years afterwards.

Should children and their family consider surgery, given the long process and the ultimate immutability of abnormal genes? One can only answer this question on a case-to-case basis. What would be the quality of life of a six-year-old who undergoes surgery, say, thirty years later? Nobody can tell. The question retains its complex answer when considering adolescents instead of younger children as well. Teenagers have a hard time following diets and often inaccurately report their attempts at weight loss. Even if they meet the physical criteria for surgery, many fail the psychological development necessary for undergoing the procedure. Consent is also an issue, with several too young to make an informed decision about undergoing an irreversible procedure. Still, bariatric surgery is generally considered an acceptable treatment for childhood and teenage obesity. Further research in the field is needed, but existing reports are clear on the fact that, if successful, bariatric surgery works brilliantly in helping patients control their weight. Non-surgical methods have been shown to be effective only in very limited capacities, and even then, patients tend to regain whatever little weight they had lost.

Who Can Get Surgery?

Not everyone who can afford bariatric surgery can get it. As has been emphasized throughout the book, surgery is a last resort, with several physical and mental factors that need to be accounted for a doctor to make a decision. The primary determinant for eligibility for surgery is BMI, which is measured using your height in meters, multiplying that number by itself, and weight in kilograms, accounting for gender. A person who has a BMI of over 30 kg/m^2 is considered obese. In 1991, the National Institutes of Health Consensus Conference approved of bariatric surgery for **adults** whose 1) BMI is above 35 kg/m^2 and are afflicted with obesity-related diseases or co-morbidities, and 2) when the BMI is above 40 kg/m^2 regardless of co-morbidity status.

The metric for qualification through a high BMI is measured differently for children and adolescents. In their case, based on the individuals' gender and age, doctors rely on the average BMI scores of a large number of children in the same age group and sex. Children's suitability for bariatric surgery is then determined based on their percentile score on the BMI. If a child weighs more than 99 per cent of all other children in their age group and who are of the same sex, they are considered eligible for surgery. This roughly translates to having a BMI of 30 kg/m^2 or above. The ninety-ninth percentile measure is used because that is the BMI where a strong positive correlation can be established between weight and high risk of cardiovascular disease.

Besides BMI, a ton of other pre-operative conditions need to be assessed for a child to qualify for surgery. As mentioned, these include a whole host of tests that analyse blood count, metabolic profile, nutrition, history of weight gain, psychiatric illness, drug/alcohol/tobacco abuse, etc. Commitment to post-operative follow-ups and lifestyle modification is also considered. Certain physical conditions *may* disqualify patients from pursuing bariatric surgery. These are: chronic pancreatitis, cirrhosis of the liver, autoimmune disease and blood disorders. Having only one of these may not make a patient ineligible for surgery, but they will require extra monitoring after surgery to minimize complications. Some conditions will immediately disqualify patients due to their significant interference with bariatric procedures. This is applicable for those who have received chemotherapy, are pregnant, suffer from Crohn's disease or from inflammatory bowel diseases.

Cost of Surgery

Speaking of those who cannot get surgery despite being able to pay for it, those who can get one, owing to their physical condition, may struggle to pay for it. This depends on where one lives, of course, but bariatric surgery is expensive regardless of the differences. India is one of the best destinations for those considering this procedure, where the cost ranges from a relatively modest Rs 2 lakh, going up to a potential Rs 7 lakh, depending on the type of procedure, and the quality of services offered. In the US, the mean cost of surgery, based on thirteen different studies, has been established as approximately USD 14,389, ranging from USD 7,400 to USD 34,000.[55] As of the day when I write this, the mean figure in dollars converts to around Rs 10 lakh, going up to roughly Rs 24 lakh. In the UK, prices range from 4,000 pounds up to 15,000 pounds, which are roughly in the range of Rs 3.5 lakh to Rs 13 lakh. The price range tends to be wide due to the variety of procedures covered under the umbrella term of 'bariatric surgery'. These types are covered in the next section.

Types of Bariatric Surgery

There are three main types of bariatric surgery: 1) Restrictive surgery, 2) Malabsorptive surgery and 3) A combination of both. Restrictive surgeries reduce the amount of food that the stomach can hold, making patients feel full faster. A normal stomach can hold around four to six cups of food, whereas after surgery, this capacity is reduced to one cup of food. Lastly, restrictive procedures include adjustable gastric banding and sleeve gastrectomy. Malabsorptive procedures involve shortening the length of the intestines, which results in fewer calories being absorbed by the body. This type of surgery was popular in the 1960s and 1970s, but the risk of severe electrolyte, nutrient and vitamin deficiencies have resulted in it falling out of favour among doctors. Three of the four currently popular surgical methods are both restrictive and malabsorptive in nature. These are gastric bypass, duodenal switch and biliopancreatic diversion. These names may sound intimidating but the next section breaks it down and explains the procedures in detail. Different procedures are suitable for different conditions, have unique success rates and the costs can drastically differ too.

All bariatric surgeries can be performed using one of two methods—the open or laparoscopic method. The primary difference between the two is the number of abdominal incisions made, which determines the exposure of internal organs. As the names suggest, an open method relies on a longer incision near the upper abdomen, whereas the laparoscopic method involves only five to six small incisions. The laparoscopic method is widely considered the safer method across all procedures due to its reduced exposure, and other technical features.

Gastric Bypass

Gastric bypass, also called Roux-en-Y gastric bypass (RYGB), is one of the two most common bariatric procedures performed across the world. As of 2011, between 40–55 per cent of all bariatric surgeries worldwide are of this type. As mentioned, malabsorptive procedures were initially the most popular form of bariatric surgery, but the risk of severe nutrient deficiencies prompted

Edward Mason to develop a technique that avoids those drawbacks. Over four decades, the procedure has evolved to become the gold standard against which all other bariatric surgeries are measured. The laparoscopic method of RYGB in particular has become popular over the last ten years due to the myriad advantages it offers. These include reduced operating time, minimal blood loss, reduced length of intensive care stay, lower post-operative pain and faster recovery.

This procedure has two major steps. In the first step, the surgeon creates a small pouch of about thirty millimetres at the top of the stomach. In the second step, the first portion of the small intestine is divided and the bottom half is attached to the newly formed stomach pouch, enabling digestion only in the smaller portion. While this may indicate that gastric bypass is merely a restrictive procedure, it does include malabsorptive mechanisms. RYGB induces favourable changes in the gut hormone levels, reduces appetite, enhances satiety and provides an environment that increases energy expenditure. Generally, lower appetite and smaller meals typically push patients to compensate by eating more meals and more calorific food. However, in what has been an unexpected result of RYGB, post-operative patients do not show this trend. This hints at it involving malabsorption as well, since fewer nutrients seem to be absorbed by the intestines.

Patients typically lose 35–40 per cent of their total body weight after RYGB, with low recidivism up to fifteen years after the procedure. This procedure also works wonders on obesity related co-morbidities. Reported rates of comorbidity resolution are: diabetes (80 per cent), hypertension (70 per cent), hypercholesterolemia (65 per cent), gastroesophageal reflux disease (75 per cent), and sleep apnoea syndrome (75 per cent). One way in which this procedure is unique is that it induces rapid weight loss after surgery as opposed to a gradual loss as seen in procedures like gastric banding. It has been argued that the increased rate might lead to nutritional deficiencies and loss of body mass. However, this rapid loss is also why RYGB is so successful in combating Type 2 diabetes, traditionally considered a progressive and unrelenting disease.

Gastric Banding

Gastric banding or Laparoscopic Gastric Banding (LAGB) is the second most popular bariatric surgery globally. About 30–45 per cent of all bariatric procedures worldwide are LAGBs. While not as successful in terms of weight loss, LAGB is the least invasive, has the lowest risk for vitamin and nutrient deficiencies and the lowest post-operative mortality rate. It also causes the least complications (most of which are minor) of all bariatric surgeries. It was developed much later than RYGB, having first been performed in 1990. Its rise in popularity can be attributed to strong celebrity endorsements and extensive media coverage.

Unlike RYGB, LAGB is reversible. Whereas RYGB is most commonly preferred in the US, where it accounts for 85 per cent of all bariatric surgeries, LAGB is more common in western Europe and Australia. This is relevant because the success rate of LAGB seems to be highly dependent on frequent post-operative follow-ups, and healthcare providers in these countries have built an efficient system to motivate this. As has been mentioned, LAGB also causes more gradual weight loss compared to the rapid loss in RYGB.

The procedure involves placing an implant—a soft silicone ring with an expandable balloon in the centre—around the top part of the stomach. It effectively divides the stomach into two pouches, with the part above the band being much smaller than the lower section. This upper part becomes the functional stomach after surgery and food consumed only fills this small pouch. LAGB is a purely restrictive procedure, since it only involves reducing an individual's stomach capacity. Patients who choose LAGB generally lose about 50–60 per cent of their excess body weight, and this weight loss remains stable for up to seven years. This number is significantly lower than that for RYGB (62 per cent), gastroplasty

(68.2 per cent), and biliopancreatic diversion (70 per cent). It is important to note that this difference is noticed for only three years after surgery has been performed, after which the rates of weight loss are virtually the same across procedures. The co-morbidity resolution rate is also lower for diabetes, with its resolution rate after surgery being 48 per cent compared to RYGBs (80 per cent), and 99 per cent for biliopancreatic diversion. For sleep apnoea disorder and hypertension, the rates are more comparable to other bariatric procedures.

LAGB is not recommended for patients who have a high risk of adverse outcomes, either due to old age or because they possess certain stomach and intestinal disorders that might interfere with the surgery. Frequent aspirin usage, alcohol and drug abuse and low commitment to post-operative follow ups and dietary modifications can also disqualify patients wishing to pursue LAGB.

Sleeve Gastrectomy

Initially, sleeve gastrectomy (SG) was used as a first step to reduce the complications associated with RYGB and biliopancreatic diversion among high-risk patients and the super obese (those who have a BMI of over 50 kg/m^2). However, the success of SG alone in helping patients lose significant amounts of weight has rendered the second step expendable. The aim of this procedure is to reduce the size of the stomach and cut off the production of a hormone called ghrelin. Ghrelin is the only known appetite stimulant and is also responsible for long-term weight regulation. Those who eat according to a fixed schedule see ghrelin levels rise automatically before meals, and a subsequent crash after eating. Average ghrelin levels also rise after weight loss. Statistics from 2013 indicate that SG is fast rising as a popular bariatric procedure, accounting for 28 per cent of all procedures worldwide, up from just 5 per cent in 2008. Despite LAGB and SG both being restrictive procedures, reduction in ghrelin levels is only observed after SG, and not after LAGB.

SG is a relatively simple procedure, involving the removal of 80–90 per cent of the patients' stomach, while the remainder has been described as resembling a 'banana' or a 'half-moon'. This is achieved by making a dissection across the stomach. The procedure is also commonly called 'partial gastrectomy', 'longitudinal gastrectomy', and 'vertical gastrectomy'. Patients lose about 50–60 per cent of their excess body weight after surgery. Like RYGB, SG has a positive effect on gut hormones that regulate hunger, satiety, and blood sugar. It reduces the amount of food consumed and improves Type 2 diabetes.

Due to its very recent popularization as a bariatric procedure, statistics on SG's short- and long- term effectiveness and risk of complications is uncertain at best. Consequently, any figures associated with such metrics must be considered with a pinch of salt. Technical variations used by doctors in the procedure also make standardization difficult, and it is unclear which technique is most beneficial. Without considering long-term data, SG has been found to provide weight loss levels at par with RYGB, but with co-morbidity resolution rates also matching RYGB rates. Diabetes was resolved in 80 per cent of all patients, hypertension in 85 per cent and 70 per cent for those with gastroesophageal reflux disease.

Biliopancreatic Diversion and Duodenal Switch

Biliopancreatic diversion with duodenal switch (BPD-DS), or simply duodenal switch, is one of the most complex and highest risk bariatric procedures one can undergo. The risk might be worth it, since it is also more effective than RYGB and LAGB. BPD-DS was first successfully performed in 1988. Along with sleeve gastrectomy, BPD-DS is a popular option for the super obese and high-risk patients. The procedure includes both restrictive and malabsorptive mechanisms. 60–70 per cent of the patients' stomach is removed, similar to the way it is done in an SG, to induce a reduced appetite. The procedure is the fourth most common bariatric surgery performed worldwide, but represents a mere 1.5 per cent of all procedures.

While in an SG, a band separates the dissected stomach from the functional one, in a BPD-DS, the stomach is stapled to create two sections. The intestine is also shortened, albeit more so than in an RYGB, leaving only a few feet of the organ for nutrient absorption. The duodenal switch is an extra step added to the BPD procedure to reduce malabsorption and ulceration, which in turn reduces the risk of nutrient deficiencies after surgery. The duodenal switch part of the procedure takes the duodenum, which is part of the small intestine connected to the stomach, and detaches it from the pylorus that is the connector between the intestines and the stomach. The ileum, which is the lower half of the intestine, is instead connected to the pylorus, effectively switching the duodenum. The duodenum is then reattached so that bile and other juices can interact with the food in the intestines. In some extreme cases, the SG part is performed first, while the BPD-DS is carried out only after a gestation period of 9–12 months.

After surgery, patients lose about 60–80 per cent of their excess body weight, and this loss remains stable for more than ten years after the procedure. Since only the super obese usually pursue BPD-DS, the weight loss percentage will be higher than procedures like RYGB and LAGB, which are more universally preferred. However, even when controlled for this variable, BPD-DS proves to be an excellent procedure for weight loss regardless of obesity level. RYGB has an impressive resolution for Type 2 diabetes (80 per cent), but BPD-DS goes one step further. It has an almost perfect record in resolving this co-morbidity in patients with a resolution rate of

98–100 per cent. A study found similarly high levels of resolution for hypertension, cholesterol, depression and gastroesophageal reflux disease. The next chapter discusses the risks associated with BPD-DS, but as surgical techniques involving this procedure evolve, these issues might well be resolved in the near future.

Endoscopic Sleeve Gastroplasty

Endoscopic sleeve gastroplasty or ESG (not to be confused with sleeve gastrectomy) is a relatively new procedure that was first successfully performed only in 2013. As such, long-term data for this procedure is unavailable. It is a minimally invasive procedure that does not require surgery.

The entire procedure only takes 2–4 hours and patients are usually discharged on the next day. The ESG reduces the volume of the stomach by approximately 40–50 per cent.

In this procedure, an endoscope is placed inside the stomach through the mouth and the walls of the stomach that need suturing are marked. A suturing device is then used to connect the walls of the stomach, which is then tightened, reducing its volume. One of the advantages of this method over LSG is that food seems to remain in the stomach for longer, making patients eat less over time. A year after surgery, patients lost around 55 per cent of their excess body weight. The immediate post-operative period can cause moderate abdominal pain or nausea, but both of these can be treated using medicines. Studies about ESG, so far, generally do not involve a lot of patients, so these results could change with research involving bigger groups. However, no long-term complications have been found to result from ESG. Like LAGB, post-operative care is a key determinant of the success of this procedure. Overall, it has been found to be a safe and effective procedure that holds much promise for the future.

Chapter 9

Life After

All surgeries involve risk. The rising popularity of bariatric surgery as an acceptable means of treatment has caused the proliferation of several procedures with varying levels of post-operative risks and complications. Obesity can cause co-morbidities in organs that start from the head (stroke, tinnitus, etc.), to those in between, such as the lungs, heart, liver, spleen, gall bladder, intestines, breasts, kidneys, legs, ovaries, right down to the toes (diabetic neuropathy, foot ulcers, etc.). That's a lot of potential diseases, and surgery could resolve or exacerbate any of them. About 10–20 per cent of patients who have bariatric surgeries require a follow-up operation to correct surgical complications. One-third of these operations are for nutritional deficiencies, such as anaemia and osteoporosis.

Even if the surgery is successful and the patient loses hundreds of pounds as a result, the miracle is sometimes not enough. New research indicates that even after years of stable weight loss patterns, patients often either return to the same destructive habits that led to their obesity, or substitute their overeating with alcoholism, drug addiction, gambling or compulsive shopping. This points to a psychological gap induced by obesity that surgery cannot cure without rigorous follow-up programmes. Obesity is a pernicious disease and has likely eroded the self-esteem of those who have suffered through it. While surgery itself might be a successful endeavour to pursue, it may not guarantee a 'happily ever after'.

Are the obese then doomed to unhappiness? It is hard to believe that one can do nothing about a condition like obesity. Adequate care, along with sustained effort on the part of the patient, are bound to help them live happily after the surgery. It is important to note that the psychological dynamics of the super obese differ from those whose obesity is less severe. The precise surgical procedure is selected based on the individuals' needs and the expertise of their doctor can also have varying effects on the psychological status of a person after surgery. There is no science that can guarantee greater mental stability in patients. However, research has thrown up some possible solutions which we will discuss ahead.

A caveat here is that these questions presuppose the safety of the procedures itself. It is of utmost importance to make the right choice regarding which surgery is best for oneself based on the associated risks, which in turn depends on the pre-operative condition of the patient. The sections below describe the various complications that might come with the different procedures outlined in the previous chapter. One thing is clear: the risks of obesity far outweigh those of bariatric surgery. Since those pursuing surgery have already been failed by therapies, such as dietary restriction, lifestyle modification and medicines, surgery is *the* last resort. Regardless of the quality of life a patient experiences after surgery, bariatric surgery is an effective option for those who have no other recourse.

Gastric Bypass

The three most prominent variables influencing complications in RYGB patients are male gender, age and severity of obesity. If a patient suffers from post-operative complications, the older they are, the more susceptible they will be to further complications and even death. Dying is extraordinarily rare in bariatric procedures in general. The mortality rate for RYGB ranges from 0–1.5 per cent. However, the list of possible complications from RYGB is a long one. It includes deep venous thrombosis, anastomotic leaks, internal hernias, gastrointestinal bleeding, ulcers in the bypassed segments, closed loop obstruction, stomal stenosis, wound complications, staple-line disruption and gallstone formation.

Of these, perhaps the most concerning is anastomotic leaks. This occurs when there are leaks of undigested food or digestive juices from the parts of the body that are reconfigured during surgery. Anastomotic leaks occurs in only about 0.7–5 per cent of patients, most of whom are super obese, but drastically increases the mortality rate of those unlucky to suffer from it. From 0–1.5 per cent, the rate rises by ten times to 15 per cent. It also increases the likelihood of contracting other complications to 61 per cent.

It is uncertain what precisely causes these leaks, but some explanations that have been offered are insufficient blood supply to the affected parts, infection, a history of smoking that inhibits post-surgical recovery and procedural errors during the surgery. Age, gender and BMI are all positively correlated to the severity of leakage. Men are more likely to contract these leaks, and older men are likelier to contract worse leaks. Common symptoms of anastomotic leaks are fever, abdominal pain, rapid heart rate and dyspnoea; these usually occur around three days after the surgery. Lastly, resolving these leaks will require further operations, either to close the leak or to make changes to accommodate it.

Short-term complication rates in RYGB are comparatively higher than other procedures. It stands at about 20 per cent for gastric bypass, 10 per cent for sleeve gastrectomy and 15 per cent for gastric banding.

Besides anastomotic leaks, other prevalent complications are internal hernias, bleeding and abdominal pain. The symptoms of many of the complications are the same as those of anastomotic leaks. It is important to note that the occurrence of complications, while potentially severe, are usually uncommon, and do not occur in more than 5–10 per cent of patients. The only exception to this rule seems to be the dumping syndrome. This syndrome occurs when chunks of food are 'dumped' directly from the stomach into the small intestine without being digested. There are two types of dumping syndrome: early and late dumping, varying in the time that the dumping takes place after eating. While the difference may seem insignificant, the symptoms for each are somewhat different. For the former, symptoms include nausea, sweating and dizziness, while the latter includes confusion, and fatigue while fainting; heart palpitations are common in both. Symptoms often disappear a year after surgery, but if needed, it can be fixed by simple dietary changes as well.

Gastric Banding

Complications with gastric banding are inevitable, but rarely life-threatening if treated properly. Approximately 50 per cent of all patients require reoperation, and 25 per cent of these occur several years after surgery. This has caused several studied patients to indicate that they would not undergo the procedure again. Common complications of LAGB are insufficient weight loss, persistent gastroesophageal reflux disease, pouch dilation, band slippage, gastric perforations, stomal obstruction and frequent vomiting. While short-term complications are rare, long-term ones are much more frequent.

Of the mentioned complications, band slippage is by far the most common. It occurs in about 80 per cent of all patients. Band slippage occurs when part of the stomach 'slips' into the functional part of the stomach, increasing its food capacity. Common symptoms of this involves a lot of vomiting. This happens either immediately or soon after eating a meal. Patients also report feeling fullness that is only resolved by regurgitation. Another symptom is pain in the upper abdomen. Severe cases of band slippage may also cause excruciating pain, increased heart rate and fever. Patients will likely need to pursue operation with one possible resolution being removing the band altogether. This is a tricky process and can result in further complications. Thankfully, doctors can drain the band of all fluid, resolving band slippage in most cases. One of the solutions scientists have come up with for problems such as band slippage is utilizing a biodegradable band so that it disappears through dissolution before symptoms worsen.

The fact that LAGB often requires reoperation, either for complications or weight recidivism, does not bode well for patients, since the risk of further complications increases with repeated surgery. Due to the associated risks, doctors are often forced to adjust their procedure to suit the patient, and often even end up performing bariatric procedures they do not have much experience with. As such, some patients experience excellent results while others are left wishing they never pursued it. Patients are also expected to make several changes in their eating habits after the operation. These include planned eating with healthy choices, careful chewing and not mixing solid and liquid food. These are key to avoiding pain and acid reflux. As has been mentioned in the previous chapter, regular follow-ups with your doctor are also key to the success of LAGB.

Sleeve Gastrectomy

Like RYGB, anastomotic leaks can be a major issue with sleeve gastrectomy. However, the characteristics of the leak from SG is different from that of RYGB. They result more commonly from SGs (about 5 per cent of all patients), and are also harder to treat due to a difference in the area where the leak occurs. Some suggested treatments are those involving fasting or placing clips to reduce the leakage. Other complications from SG include haemorrhage, persistent gastroesophageal reflux disease, nutritional deficiencies, abdominal abscess, stricture, pulmonary embolism and wound infections.

In the long term, SG has several benefits over RYGB and LAGB. It avoids complications like hernia, usage of foreign objects such as bands, and the intestines are not interfered with since SG is purely restrictive in nature.

This renders it more treatable through endoscopies. Furthermore, dumping syndrome and ulceration are highly uncommon after the SG. Due to the relatively recent rise of SG as a viable bariatric procedure, data on weight recidivism or insufficient weight loss forcing re-operation is unavailable.

Besides leaks, pulmonary embolism is another potentially catastrophic complication arising from SG. This is a condition wherein one or more arteries in the lungs are blocked by a blood clot. Pulmonary embolism is observed in RYGB patients as well, and most research only tracks embolism in that procedure. Hence, more study is needed before making any claims about embolisms after the SG, but it has been reported, and could be a fatal complication for SG patients.

A third potentially fatal complication arising from SG is venous thromboembolism (VTE). This condition arises when a blood clot is formed in the veins around the legs, groin and arms. While the probability of contracting thromboembolism is quite low, it can result in death. Those undergoing reoperation, long bariatric procedures or those with a very high BMI are all at risk of suffering from VTE. Chances of VTE are exacerbated if the patient is male, a smoker and has a history of VTE. Besides patient-related factors, the nature of the procedure might cause further complications, such as if the surgery is open or laparoscopic (see previous chapter), and the presence of anastomotic leaks as a result of faulty surgical methods. Overall, while the occurrence of complications from SG is low, the ones that do occur can be a cause for concern.

Duodenal Switch

In the previous chapter, biliopancreatic diversion with duodenal switch (BPD-DS) was stated to be the most effective bariatric procedure for weight loss, which tends to remain stable for more than a decade after surgery. The flipside is that it is also the most technically complex surgery of all available treatments. This procedure has about three to four steps, and each step takes a few hours to complete. The longer the procedure, the higher the risk of complications. The post-operative mortality rate of patients who pursued BPD-DS is the highest of all bariatric procedures, ranging from 0.29–1.23 per cent for open procedures, and 0–2.7 per cent for laparoscopic ones. One possible explanation for this could be that BPD-DS is safer for the super obese compared to other procedures. This group has the highest risk of complications after surgery, and so mortality rates for this procedure are higher than the rest. In a study of 700 patients, about 5 per cent of them needed corrective surgery for surgical complications.

Some of the most common risks associated with BPD-DS have already been discussed. These include bleeding, duodenal leakage, anastomotic leaks and venous thromboembolism. The DS part of the BPD-DS can cause severe nutritional, protein and vitamin deficiencies, along with diarrhoea and other rectal complications. This occurs because the length of the bowel is shortened during the duodenal switch. Other risks include nausea, loose stools, heartburn, vomiting, constipation and bloating. Most BPD-DS patients experience at least a few of these in some capacity either on a daily, weekly or monthly basis. However, it is important to note that these symptoms are common amongst RYGB patients as well.

Should One Get Surgery?

In one word, the answer is yes. This chapter has attempted to detail the various complications associated with various procedures, and some of them can be fatal. But as has been mentioned, the risks of remaining morbidly obese are much greater than those of bariatric surgery. Most, if not all people who undergo surgery, will likely suffer from either minor complications like vomiting, diarrhoea, constipation, etc., or major ones like leaks, venous or pulmonary embolism, and stricture. Minor complications can usually be treated with medical therapy of some form, and the major ones are extraordinarily rare. Even then, they seldom result in death, and can be treated with proper care. Bariatric surgery has also been pursued for those primarily suffering from Type 2 diabetes, even among the non-obese. A systematic review conducted in 2014 concluded that across bariatric procedures, complications occur in 10–17 per cent of patients and reoperation rates stand at approximately

7 per cent. The mortality associated with bariatric surgery is about 0.08–0.35 per cent.

Psychological and Behavioural Aftercare

Often, the massive weight loss resulting from bariatric surgery is not enough to improve the quality of life of patients. Women who lost tons of weight after surgery noticed significant improvements in the predisposition of people towards them. People are friendlier, warmer and listen with greater interest when these women speak. This can be quite provocative, since many find it unfair that they had to undergo weight loss for their acquaintances to treat them better. They also express disappointment at the stigma that still surrounds obesity. This results in many explaining their weight loss as having been achieved by undergoing hard dietary programmes rather than admitting that they pursued corrective surgery.

As mentioned, recidivism rates are high, even years after the surgery has been performed. Furthermore, many replace the compulsive eating habits that led to their obesity with other toxic habits such as gambling, substance abuse, etc. Up to 70 per cent of all bariatric patients suffer from some form of mental health illness pre-surgery, and this is a large reason why psychological assessment is a key practice among doctors determining suitable candidates for surgery. However, the guidelines for psychiatric care after illness lack uniformity or consensus. Some surgeons have suggested that patients' unique psychological profiles need to be incorporated into the structure of pre- and post-operative care. This section discusses the different courses of action that patients can adopt to maximize the benefits they are sure to attain from surgery, and to improve general happiness. It also highlights the structure of psychological assessment before surgery, and how that impacts recovery after the procedure.

It is important to emphasize again that significant gaps exist in regard to research about psychological well-being after surgery. A 2018 study claims that this metric has not been studied beyond twenty-four months after surgery, which is the period when weight regain is most common. There is no evidence to suggest that pre-operative psychiatric illness has any significant impact on surgical effectiveness. The same 2018 study also concluded that patients who had undergone counselling after surgery had similar mental well-being scores as compared to those who had not. Decrease in mental health issues, such as anxiety and depression, have also been observed up to a year after surgery. This is the period when most of the weight loss from bariatric procedures occurs, making the previous observation an intuitive one. However, studies have shown that psychological assessments have consistently showed improved scores for up to ten years after surgery, despite weight loss rates reducing after the one year mark

While one would assume that bariatric procedures would have more or less the same effect on psychological well-being, this does not seem to be the case. It has been found that those who pursued the sleeve gastrectomy procedure are three times more likely to pursue counselling than those who chose gastric banding. A distinction needs to be made between those whose BMI is over 50 kg/m^2 and those between 40–50 kg/m^2. While neither group is likely to suffer from serious psychological issues, such as schizophrenia or bipolar disorder, up to 95 per cent of morbidly obese patients have reported issues such as anxiety, depression, denial, loneliness, general distrust and somatization. This is a huge number and lends greater credence to the argument that one's psychological profile needs to be factored into bariatric treatment.

There is also the case of surgical complications being mistaken for psychological issues. For example, frequent vomiting is a common consequence of surgery. This symptom reduces with time, but is sometimes confused with bulimia or other eating disorders. Conversely, it is possible that some patients self-induce vomiting beyond the usual timeframe of its occurrence for sustained weight loss. As such, despite the high frequency of such symptoms in patients, they may need to be monitored to ensure their safety and good health.

Another worrying trend relating to psychological well-being is that anti-depressant usage does not seem to decrease in any significant way after surgery. Two studies have suggested that only 9 per cent and 16 per cent patients reduce their psychotropic medication. This is in contrast with the dramatic reduction in medication for serious physical diseases such as diabetes mellitus (76 per cent), hypertension (51 per cent) and hyperlipidaemia (59 per cent). The type of procedure one chooses can have significant effects on this. Malabsorptive procedures like gastric bypass can pose issues for dissolution of medicines, demanding a switch in medicines, which could be dangerous, or even lead to an increase in dosage.

Psychological Evaluation Before Surgery

Psychological evaluation before the surgery usually involves a clinical interview and psychological testing to determine a variety of factors such as bariatric knowledge, adherence, eating behaviours, mood, substance use, cognitive functioning and history of mental health.

Eating behaviours are assessed along three major patterns: binge, night time and emotional eating. These patterns can lead to vomiting, constipation and dumping syndrome after surgery. Binge eating is defined as eating an excessive amount of food in a short period of time. Associated factors can include secretive eating, eating until uncomfortably full and guilt about overeating. As many as 52 per cent of those seeking surgery suffer from this disorder. It can be said that one is eating too much at night if over 25 per cent of one's calorie intake occurs after evening, along with waking up at night solely to eat, at least twice a week. This is rarer than binge eating, occurring in only about 1.5 per cent of patients and can cause issues with metabolism. Lastly, emotional eating, as the name suggests, is the overconsumption of food as a response to stress-inducing stimuli. Eating disorders have only been classified as mental disorders in the most recent edition of the *Diagnostic and Statistic Manual for Mental Disorders* (DSM-V). As such, diagnostic criteria for these illnesses are unclear. Some solutions that have been offered include encouraging patients to maintain a food diary to track their eating patterns for a certain period before surgery. Electronic monitoring devices are available in the market to help in this endeavour, along with apps accessible through smartphones. Specific behavioural recommendations are also important in helping patients replace their old patterns. These can vary widely, and can only be provided on the basis of individual assessments.

With regard to psychological testing and interviewing, truthfulness is a major issue since these tests often ask deeply personal questions relating to suicidal tendencies, sexual abuse and other embarrassing details that the patient may never have spoken to anyone about. One can hardly blame patients for wanting to lie, given its convenience and the difficulty associated with articulating feelings, especially for people who are highly susceptible to anxiety and depression. In my own research, several sites appeared to offer 'tricks' to help one pass the rounds of psychological testing that bariatric patients compulsorily need to undergo. Surprisingly, most of them advise patients to be honest. In an interview, a surgeon emphasized that regular testing over time can be used to judge the consistency of patients' answers.

Some criteria that may exclude patients from receiving surgery are: 1) an active psychosis, or cognitive impairment that may interfere with the patients' ability to adhere to post-operative behaviour changes, 2) hospitalization for the psychosis within the last year, 3) multiple suicide attempts in the last five years, 4) evidence of an alcohol or substance use disorder in the last five months, 5) unstable social environment (homelessness, lack of access to a kitchen), 6) low scores on self-motivation or personal responsibility as determined by specific tests. Disqualification is not the end, however, and correcting whichever factor caused the ineligibility through therapy can allow one to pursue bariatric surgery in the future.

Psychological Care after Surgery

One of the most critical elements of post-operative mental healthcare is the involvement of a team of professionals rather than a single psychologist in combating issues holistically. This is deemed to encourage greater communication and focuses on issues, such as nutrition as well. Interviews have revealed that many patients do not attempt weight loss in any rigorous manner before surgery, and even if they do, they are usually short-lived and ineffective. This relates to the attitudes of patients who perceive surgery as the final solution to their problems, but as has been discussed, this is far from the case. A team of professionals can thus build psycho-educational programmes that are unique to individuals, and help them overcome these false beliefs.

It was earlier mentioned that patients experience significant improvements in mental health up to a year after the procedure. This was attributed to rapid weight loss in the same period. However, a reputable study of 4,000 obese patients has found that in many cases, surgery acted as a catalyst for patients who had a renewed interest in improving their physical condition. This occurred even in cases where weight loss from surgery was less than expected. Despite this, the report maintains that a considerable minority do face issues coping with their new bodies. Some face issues like loose skin after the procedure, which continues to pose a hindrance to their self-esteem, while others are disturbed by the increasing warmth of colleagues and friends simply due to their weight loss.

Afterword

It is often assumed that the end goal of surgery is weight loss. But as cited in the beginning of the book, the journey and relationship with one's weight is attributed to many aspects.

Beyond health and nutrition, food is intertwined with social parameters, emotional well-being, celebrations, expressing love and concern and so on. Hence, even weight loss and maintenance should pave the way for a sustainable and balanced life while enjoying tasty but nutritious food for nourishment. This is imperative for the individual to live a content, healthy and fulfilled life, which has probably become possible after undergoing surgery.

Surgery and psychological care after surgery should allow the patient to adopt a way of life that furthers the positive aspects of weight loss rather than looking at weight loss as the ultimate objective. Weight loss and a healthy weight are tools to live a comfortable and healthy life that allows you to function efficiently and live life to the fullest.

That, my dear patients, is perhaps the end goal of this book and my attempt to help you to live to your optimum potential, aided by a healthy mind and body.

Acknowledgements

There have been many challenges in my life, right from my MBBS years, post-graduation to twenty-five years of practice as a surgeon. To enumerate those countless interesting cases was almost impossible. However, this herculean task was taken upon by Gurveen Chaddha. She has been relentlessly persistent right from the inception of the idea.

The other motivational individual was my dear friend Santosh Andhale. His vast experience in the field as a health journalist was immensely helpful and encouraging for an amateur like me.

Malathi Iyer, another stalwart health Journalist from Times of India, took upon the role of a wise sensei. A sincere thanks to one of our consultants, 'Mom' Nisha Nair. Like Robin and Batman, they were a fantastic duo, and I enjoyed our many meetings in the making of the book. I am forever indebted.

And, of course, words fail me when I come to my home team.

My wife Sandhya's support and her untiring attitude which was infectious in those dark and dreary days. She was just the medication I needed and more.

Lastly my son, my apprentice, my colleague, Dr Rahul, was very helpful in compiling and gathering the data.

My beautiful and smart daughter Mitali's humorous quips and banter broadened my smile on the most tiresome days. Thank you all for being on my ringside.